Type 2 Diabetes for Beginners 2nd Edition

A user-friendly guide on taking the right steps toward a healthy life with diabetes

Phyllis Barrier, MS

American Diabetes Association.

Director, Book Publishing, Abe Ogden; *Acquisitions Editor*, Victor Van Beuren; *Editor*, Greg Guthrie, *Production Manager*, Melissa Sprott; *Composition*, ADA; *Cover Design*, Vis-à-Vis Creative Concepts; *Printer*, United Graphics, Inc.

Printed in the United States of America
3 5 7 9 10 8 6 4 2

The suggestions and information contained in this publication are generally consistent with the Clinical Practice Recommendations and other policies of the American Diabetes Association, but they do not represent the policy or position of the Association or any of its boards or committees. Reasonable steps have been taken to ensure the accuracy of the information presented. However, the American Diabetes Association cannot ensure the safety or efficacy of any product or service described in this publication. Individuals are advised to consult a physician or other appropriate health care professional before undertaking any diet or exercise program or taking any medication referred to in this publication. Professionals must use and apply their own professional judgment, experience, and training and should not rely solely on the information contained in this publication before prescribing any diet, exercise, or medication. The American Diabetes Association—its officers, directors, employees, volunteers, and members—assumes no responsibility or liability for personal or other injury, loss, or damage that may result from the suggestions or information in this publication.

♾ The paper in this publication meets the requirements of the ANSI Standard Z39.48-1992 (permanence of paper).

ADA titles may be purchased for business or promotional use or for special sales. To purchase more than 50 copies of this book at a discount, or for custom editions of this book with your logo, contact the American Diabetes Association at the address below, at booksales@diabetes.org, or by calling 703-299-2046.

American Diabetes Association
1701 North Beauregard Street
Alexandria, Virginia 22311

DOI: 10.2337/9781580404426

Library of Congress Cataloging-in-Publication Data

Barrier, Phyllis, 1946-
  Type 2 diabetes for beginners / Phyllis Barrier. -- 2nd ed.
     p. cm.
  Includes bibliographical references and index.
  ISBN 978-1-58040-442-6 (pbk.)
  1. Non-insulin-dependent diabetes--Popular works. I. Title. II. Title: Type two diabetes for beginners.
  RC662.18.B37 2011
  616.4'624--dc23
                    2011017907

*To the people with diabetes
who have taught me so much
about combining life and diabetes care.*

*To my parents
and to my husband, Michael.*

Contents

Foreword ix
Acknowledgments xiii
Introduction 1

Chapter

1   What Is Prediabetes? 5

2   Type 1 and Type 2 Diabetes:
What's the Difference? 9

3   Eating with Prediabetes or Type 2 Diabetes 13
Rate Your Plate 14
Carbohydrate Counting 16
Steps in Using a Food Label 26
Making Healthy Food Choices 28
Glycemic Index 31
Using Meal Planning Tools 32

4   Meal Planning and Shopping 37

5   Tips for Eating Out with Diabetes 45
Top Tips for Eating Away from Home 46

6 What to Eat When You're Sick 49
Tips for Sick Days 49
Liquid and Soft Sick Day Foods 50
When to Call Your Health Care Team 52

7 Checking Your Blood Glucose 57
Using a Blood Glucose Meter 58
How Often Do I Check My Blood Glucose? 59
The A1C or eAG Check 61

8 Keeping Your Blood Glucose
in Your Target Range 65

9 What Makes Your Blood Glucose
Go Up or Down? 67
If Your Blood Glucose Is Too High 70
What Can I Do When My Blood Glucose Is High? . . .71
If Your Blood Glucose Is Too Low 72
What Can I Do When My Blood Glucose Is Too Low? .73

10 Get Up and Get Going 77
Get Ready to Be More Active 80
Get Set 81
Go for It: Making a Plan and Getting Started 82
Go for It! 85

11 Guidelines for Diabetes Care 87
At Every Diabetes Visit 88
At Least Twice a Year 89
Every Year 89
Things to Do before Each Diabetes Visit 90
Taking Charge of Your Diabetes Visits 92

12 Diabetes Medicines 95
What Kind of Pill Is It? 96
Injectable Diabetes Medications 100
Insulin 100

Insulin Shots. 103
Taking Your Medicines 109

13 Do You Want to Lose Weight?. 113
Ways to Lose Weight. 114
Knowing When You're Ready to Lose Weight 123
Making Your Plan to Lose Weight 123
How to Track Your Progress. 125

14 Diabetes and Depression 127
Signs of Depression. 128
How Is Depression Treated? 131
Your Risk for Depression. 132

15 Stress and Diabetes. .133
Are You Stressed Out? 135
Dealing with Stress 136

16 Smoking and Diabetes 139
Double Trouble 139
Are You Ready to Quit Smoking? 141
Making a Plan 141

17 Sex and Diabetes. 147
For Men Only. 147
For Women Only. 149
Pregnancy and Diabetes 150
Birth Control and Diabetes. 152

18 Alcohol and Diabetes 153
Guidelines for Drinking Alcohol
with Type 2 Diabetes. 153

19 Long-Term Diabetes Problems 157
Eye Problems. 159
Foot Problems 161
Heart and Blood Vessel Problems. 165
Kidney Problems 174

Nerve Problems 176
Skin Problems 178
Tooth and Gum Problems 180
Diabetes Problems: Putting It All Together 183

20 What It All Means 185

21 Diabetes Tools 189
Carbohydrate Choices 189
My Blood Glucose Log 194
My Medicines 195
My Meal Plan 196
My Shopping List 198
Resources 201

Index 203

Foreword

by Barbara Anderson

When we read a book, we read "within the lines" and "between the lines." "Within the lines" means that we pay attention to what the author has written, to the printed facts and the information. "Between the lines" refers to both the emotional tone in which the facts and information are given as well as the information that the author has not included. *Type 2 Diabetes for Beginners*, which has been written by a seasoned nutritionist with substantial diabetes experience, has the comprehensive information and facts "within" its lines— from carb counting to stress management—that a person needs in order to begin and maintain a life with diabetes. However, what is most unique about this book is that it also communicates "between the lines," providing the essential emotional message that it takes determination, courage, and support to maintain the stamina to sustain this journey in living with diabetes. The experienced nutritionist who wrote

Type 2 Diabetes for Beginners is also an experienced clinician and has worked for years with individuals with diabetes and their families. Phyllis Barrier understands that what patients and families need does not simply end at the information and facts, but also requires energy, optimism, and engagement to successfully apply diabetes facts and create and continue healthy lifestyle changes.

As to information that is not included in this book, you will find no mention of how easy it is to live with diabetes. You will not find misleading messages that say you can "do it all yourself." In fact, you are assured that living with diabetes is a difficult challenge and that everyone on the road needs two teams—an experienced health care team and a family/friend support team. What I appreciate most about this book is its honest and reassuring tone. Within the lines and between them, the person with diabetes is guided to take small and realistic steps to create and continue needed lifestyle changes. And as Phyllis has said so strongly within and between the lines, building a long and healthy life with diabetes can be a realistic long-term goal for everyone with diabetes.

Barbara Anderson, PhD
Professor, Pediatric Endocrinology and Metabolism
Baylor College of Medicine
Houston, Texas

by Martha M. Funnell

I am honored to introduce this book and congratulate you on taking this important step in caring for your diabetes. If you are like many of the people whom I see as a diabetes educator and you just found out that you have type 2 diabetes, you are probably feeling somewhat overwhelmed. You may also be feeling angry, scared, or confused.

You probably also have questions. You may have concerns about taking care of a chronic illness such as diabetes. And you may have discovered that diabetes is different from other illnesses you have had. Having diabetes means that there are many decisions to be made each day about how you care for yourself. Making wise choices will make a difference in both how you feel today and your future health.

You may also want to begin to make some changes in your life that will help you take better care of yourself and your diabetes. As much as you truly want to make these changes, it is never easy, especially when it comes to how you eat, handle stress, and exercise.

It may help to know that you are not alone. This book is written to be a resource to help you learn how to manage and cope with diabetes. You may not know a lot about diabetes yet, but you do know about yourself and what is important to you. When you combine what you know with what your health care team knows about diabetes, you'll have a powerful combination.

I often tell my patients that diabetes is a journey. It is probably not a journey that you would have chosen, and it is not an easy one. But even the hardest journey is made easier when you can lighten your load. This book can be a guide for you. The more you know, the more you will feel that you are in charge of diabetes, rather than allowing diabetes to control you. You can also learn how to make decisions that are right for you and make changes in your life so that you not only live long but live well.

Best wishes on your journey.

Martha M. Funnell, MS, RN, CDE
Michigan Diabetes Research and Training Center
Ann Arbor, Michigan

Acknowledgments

Len Boswell, former Vice President, Publications, American Diabetes Association, came up with the idea for a book that would help people who are just beginning to deal with type 2 diabetes, whether newly diagnosed or just starting to care for their long-standing diabetes. I am grateful that he asked me to write it.

Many other staff members at the National Office of the American Diabetes Association helped make this book a reality. Special thanks to Abe Ogden, Director of Book Publishing; Greg Guthrie, Managing Editor; Stephanie Dunbar, MPh, RD, Director of Nutrition and Medical Affairs; and the illustrators and graphic designers.

Thanks also to the many volunteers I worked with at the American Diabetes Association. They taught me so much through the years. I cannot possibly list them all, but I hope they know who they are! I do want to single out those volunteers who worked with me on the Program Publications

Editorial Board: Martha M. Funnell, MS, RN, CDE; Virginia Paragallo-Dittko, MA, RN, CDE; Barbara Anderson, PhD; Patricia Barr, BS; Carol Homko, PhD, RN, CDE; Melinda Maryniuk, MEd, RD, CDE; Catherine Mullooly, MS, CDE; Robin Nwankwo, MPH, RD, CDE; Cecilia Boyer Casey, MS, RN, CDE; Richard Rubin, PhD, CDE; and Andrea Zaldivar, MS, ANP, CDE. Marion Franz, MS, RD, CDE, and Madelyn Wheeler, MS, RD, were my wonderful diabetes and nutrition mentors who always had time for a question or volunteer project.

And last, but not least, I want to thank my parents for their sacrifices and support through the years. I also want to thank my husband, Michael, who has been my best friend, sounding board, and "at-home editor."

Introduction

Diabetes has been part of my life for many years. You see, diabetes is in my family. My Aunt Carla has had diabetes for as long as I can remember. My cousin Pam has had diabetes for a number of years. Other cousins have now been diagnosed with prediabetes or type 2 diabetes. I guess you can say that diabetes runs in my family. My mom has type 2 diabetes, too. A number of my high school friends now have type 2 diabetes. Many people I love have diabetes. Many people you love probably have prediabetes or type 2 diabetes, too. And you or a family member or friend may have been told you have prediabetes or type 2 diabetes. Since writing the first edition of this book five years ago, my circle of family, friends, colleagues, and neighbors with prediabetes or type 2 diabetes has grown substantially. You see, diabetes is an epidemic in our country. Close to 2 million adults are diagnosed with diabetes each year.

As a Registered Dietitian (RD), I worked for 30 years with people who have diabetes. I was a Certified Diabetes Educator (CDE) for 20 years. A CDE is a health care provider who specializes in diabetes education. I had to pass a special exam. I have worked in health departments with kids, adults, and pregnant women who had diabetes. I have worked in managed care, helping people learn how to take care of their diabetes.

I most recently worked at the National Office for the American Diabetes Association for more than 11 years. I helped write guidelines and booklets for people with prediabetes and type 2 diabetes. I am lucky enough to still be developing and writing educational materials for them as a consultant.

The American Diabetes Association asked me to write this book in 2005 and to update this edition in 2011. The American Diabetes Association has many fine books, but they wanted me to write a book that focuses on the basic stuff— what you really need to know if you've recently been diagnosed with prediabetes or type 2 diabetes. Many people I've worked with through the years have told me, "My life is too busy as it is. Just tell me what I need to do to take care of my diabetes." Well, here it is.

If you've recently been diagnosed with prediabetes or type 2 diabetes, you may be scared. Or you may have had diabetes for a while but haven't taken care of it. Too much glucose in the blood for a long time can cause diabetes problems. If you've been told you have a diabetes problem, you may be scared, too. This book will be helpful whether you've been recently diagnosed or have had diabetes for a while. You may know about the problems that diabetes has caused your family or friends. But you may not have heard the **good news** about having prediabetes or type 2 diabetes today:

- You can have a healthy, active, and long life with prediabetes or type 2 diabetes.
- You can learn to cope with the ups and downs of living with prediabetes or type 2 diabetes.
- You can take care of yourself by using a meal plan, being active most days of the week, and taking diabetes medicines, if needed.
- If you have prediabetes, you can delay or prevent getting type 2 diabetes.
- You can delay or prevent long-term problems by caring for your diabetes each day.

When it comes to your diabetes care, the experts agree that you're in charge. Sure, you go to the doctor or see a nurse educator every few months. But you choose what and how much to eat. You decide whether you'll take your diabetes medicine, check your blood glucose, and be active.

You're in charge, but you're not alone. Lean on your diabetes team for care and support. Who is on your diabetes team? It might be your spouse, your partner, your kids, your parents, your friends, or other members of your family. It might be a neighbor you've known for years. It might be people from your church or synagogue or from where you work. Your diabetes health care team can include your doctor, diabetes educator, dietitian, eye doctor, foot doctor, and mental health counselor.

Many of the people on your team may also have diabetes. Today many people in the United States and around the world have diabetes. Almost 26 million children and adults in the United States have diabetes. Seventy-nine million more have prediabetes.

There's never a vacation from having diabetes or caring for your diabetes. But as millions of people know, you can live a healthy and happy life with it.

Turn to the table of contents to start learning how. From the list of chapters, you can choose where to start. You may want to zoom to Chapter 7 to learn more about checking blood glucose. Or you may want to start with Chapter 3 and go on to 4, 5, and 6. They deal with food and diabetes. Or you may just want to start at the beginning and read through the book. It's your choice!

—1—

What Is Prediabetes?

Prediabetes is a condition that comes before type 2 diabetes. It means that blood glucose (GLOO-kos) levels are higher than normal but aren't high enough to be called diabetes. As we become older, or less active, or gain weight, we are more at risk for prediabetes and type 2 diabetes. People can have prediabetes and not know it.

If you have prediabetes, it means:

- you might get type 2 diabetes sometime soon or further down the road.
- you are more likely to get heart disease or have a stroke.

The good news is that you can take steps to delay or prevent type 2 diabetes with:

- weight loss
- regular physical activity, such as walking almost every day

A study called the Diabetes Prevention Program showed that these steps helped most people delay or prevent type 2 diabetes. Losing weight and being active worked well for people of all ages.

Weight loss can delay or prevent type 2 diabetes. Reaching a healthy weight can help you a lot. If you're overweight, any weight loss, even 10 or 15 pounds, will lower your chances of getting type 2 diabetes.

Losing extra weight helped people in the Diabetes Prevention Program delay or prevent type 2 diabetes. People in the study lost an average of 15 pounds in the first year of the study. How did they do it? They ate fewer calories and less fat. And they exercised most days of the week. In fact, many walked about 150 minutes a week.

Being active almost every day is another one of the best ways to delay or prevent type 2 diabetes. You can lower your chances of getting type 2 diabetes by adding physical activity to your daily routine. Even if you have heart disease or other problems, you can still be more active. Work with your health care team to find out which physical activities are safe for you.

As we all know, losing weight and getting active can be hard. And sticking with it can be even harder. The American Diabetes Association suggests an ongoing support group and counseling to help. Diabetes medicines may be added if you're at high risk for getting type 2.

It helps to keep track of the progress you're making with eating and walking. Write down everything you eat and drink for a week. Writing things down makes you more aware of what you're eating and helps with weight loss. You can keep track of your walking by wearing a pedometer on your belt. A pedometer is a small device that tells you how many steps you've taken. Or you can keep track of your walking or other activity by writing it down for a week. At the end of the week, total up the minutes you've been active to see how you're doing.

If you have prediabetes, you may suspect that someone you love has prediabetes or type 2 diabetes. At their next doctor visit, ask them to get their blood glucose checked if they are:

- 45 or older
- Under 45, but overweight and have one or more of these risk factors:

  - They have a close family member, like a parent, brother, or sister, with diabetes.
  - They are:
    - African American
    - Native American
    - Asian American
    - Pacific Islander
    - Hispanic American (Latino)

  - They've had a baby weighing more than nine pounds or they've had gestational (jess-TAY-shuhn-uhl) diabetes. Gestational diabetes is diabetes first found during pregnancy that is not type 1 or type 2.
  - They have high blood pressure (over 140/90) or are taking a blood pressure medication.

- They have low HDL cholesterol, the good cholesterol (35 or lower).
- They have high triglycerides (250 or higher).

Small steps lead to big rewards. Taking small steps to change the way you eat and increase your activity can delay or prevent type 2 diabetes. Decide how you'll reduce your calories to lose weight. Think about what you're willing and able to do to be more active almost every day.

Type 2 diabetes is a serious disease. If you delay or prevent it, you'll enjoy better health in the long run. Feeling good and having energy are keys to living the good life.

—2—

Type 1 and Type 2 Diabetes: What's the Difference?

There are many types of diabetes, but the two most common are type 1 and type 2 diabetes. Diabetes means that your blood glucose is too high.

Everyone's blood has some sugar in it because your body needs sugar for energy. Our brain can only work if it has blood glucose. But too much glucose in your blood—too much sugar—can mean you have diabetes. Normally, your body breaks food down into glucose and sends it into your

Blood Sugar vs. Blood Glucose

You may have heard people talk about their sugar when they talk about diabetes. Your doctor or another member of your diabetes health care team may talk to you about blood sugar or blood glucose. Blood sugar and blood glucose are the same. In this book, I'll use blood glucose when talking about the amount of sugar or glucose in your blood.

bloodstream. Then your pancreas (PAN-kree-us) makes a hormone called insulin (IN-suh-lin). Insulin's job is to help get the glucose from the blood into your body's cells, where it can be used for energy. Insulin helps keep blood glucose in a normal range.

In type 1 diabetes, the pancreas makes little or no insulin. People with type 1 diabetes get insulin from a shot or a pump to keep their blood glucose in their target range. Most people with type 1 diabetes take two to four shots a day or use an insulin pump. Old names for type 1 diabetes are juvenile-onset diabetes or insulin-dependent diabetes. Type 1 diabetes is not as common as type 2 diabetes.

People with prediabetes or type 2 diabetes still make insulin. But their pancreas may not be making enough, or their body may not be using it the right way. People with prediabetes or type 2 diabetes can manage their condition by watching what they eat, by being more active, and sometimes by taking diabetes medicines. Old names for type 2 diabetes are "maturity-onset diabetes" or "adult-onset diabetes," but now kids are getting type 2. Type 2 diabetes is the most common type of diabetes.

Kids who are overweight and aren't active are more likely to get prediabetes or type 2 diabetes. So are kids who have a family member with diabetes. Some racial and ethnic groups have a greater risk of getting diabetes: Native Americans, African Americans, Hispanic Americans (Latinos), Asian Americans, and Pacific Islanders.

Today everyone knows someone who has diabetes. It may be a family member, like your mother, your aunt, or your child. Or it may be a coworker or good friend. When I worked for the American Diabetes Association, I always carried my American Diabetes Association work bag when I traveled on an airplane. Every single time, someone on the plane would talk to me about diabetes. They talked about their grandchild's diabetes, about their brother's diabetes, or about their own diabetes.

Diabetes is serious, and more people are getting it. By taking care of your diabetes and showing others how to do it, you may prevent people you love from getting diabetes. You can be a role model for people around you.

People with type 1 or type 2 diabetes do some of the same things to care for their diabetes. They watch what they eat, they are active, and they check their blood glucose levels using a meter. But we'll learn more about all of that in later chapters in this book.

—3—

Eating with Prediabetes or Type 2 Diabetes

When people find out they have prediabetes or type 2 diabetes, the first thing they want to know is what they can eat, when they can eat, and how much they can eat. In fact, studies show that people with diabetes find dealing with food the hardest part of their diabetes care.

Many people think that having diabetes means they can't eat their favorite foods. But that's just not true. You can still eat the foods you love. By working with your dietitian and by reading this book, you will know how to include your favorite foods and still keep your blood glucose levels on track. For more information on blood glucose goals, see Chapter 8.

For most of us, food means more than just getting full. Eating meals brings us together with family and friends. It brings comfort and pleasure. That's why, for most people with diabetes, food is the toughest part. There's no doubt about it. Changing the way you eat or the times you eat can be really tough. But keep in mind that you're in charge—you can do it.

When you're first told you have prediabetes or type 2 diabetes, you may not be able to meet with a dietitian right away. So what do you do? There are many ways to take on diabetes meal planning, so let's talk about some of those ways. The first diabetes meal planning method I'll talk about is called Rate Your Plate.

Rate Your Plate

Life isn't easy, and having diabetes isn't easy. But an easy first step in meal planning is to Rate Your Plate. With prediabetes and type 2 diabetes, the amount of food you eat affects your blood glucose. Rate Your Plate is a method that helps you judge your food portions. In fact, Rate Your Plate gives you portion power. For most people with prediabetes or type 2 diabetes, eating smaller portions makes their blood glucose go down. Here's how Rate Your Plate works. After you've put your food on your plate, take a look:

- Is about one-fourth of your plate filled with starchy foods, such as noodles, rice, corn, peas, or potatoes?

- Is about one-fourth of your plate filled with main dish (protein) foods, like meat, poultry, fish, or meat substitutes, such as cheese, eggs, or tofu?

- Is at least half of your plate filled with cooked or raw vegetables, such as salad, or cooked vegetables like carrots, green beans, spinach, or sliced tomatoes?

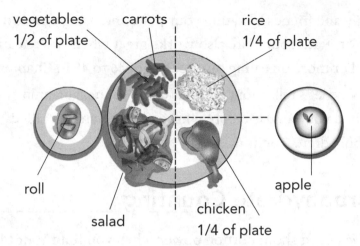

vegetables
1/2 of plate

carrots

rice
1/4 of plate

roll

apple

salad

chicken
1/4 of plate

- You may also want to add one or two side foods along with your meal, such as a dinner roll and a small piece of fruit.

Check your plate against the picture shown above. How did you do? What changes do you think you need to make?

- Do you need to work on including more vegetables or fruit?
- Do you need to cut back on starches?

☞ I'll work on _____ this week.

Now you know how to Rate Your Plate. Other members of your family who don't have diabetes but want to lose weight might want to rate their plates along with you. Your family is a key part of your diabetes team when it comes to food and meal planning. Lean on them. Ask them for help and support. You may also become a role model for your family and friends by rating your plate and using **portion power**. Rate Your Plate also works great when you're eating out. For more on eating out, see pages 46 to 48 in Chapter 5.

Now let's talk about another diabetes meal planning method you can use before you see a dietitian. It's called Carbohydrate Counting.

Carbohydrate Counting

We've talked about portion power when you Rate Your Plate. Now we're going to talk about **portion power** with a focus on carbohydrates.

Carbohydrate counting is also called by a shorter name, Carb Counting. By counting carbohydrates, or carbs, in the foods you eat, you'll have another way to keep your blood glucose on track. All foods contain the nutrients that your body needs: carbohydrate, protein, and fat.

- **Carbohydrate.** Carbohydrate foods can be put into four groups:

  1. Starches, such as crackers, cereal, corn, bread, rice, and tortillas
  2. Fruits, such as apples, berries, cherries, mangos, and peaches
  3. Milk products, such as milk, yogurt, or buttermilk
  4. Sweets and desserts, such as cookies, cake, ice cream, and pastries. Some sugar-free and fat-free foods have carbohydrate, too.

- **Protein.** Protein foods can be put into two groups:

1. Meats, such as beef, pork, fish, or chicken
2. Meat substitutes, such as beans, cheese, eggs, or tofu

- **Fat.** Fats can be divided into four groups:

    1. Unsaturated fats are found in canola oil, olive oil, avocado, and nuts like almonds and walnuts. They can protect your heart by lowering your blood cholesterol.
    2. Saturated fats are found in high-fat meats, such as hot dogs, sausage, and in high-fat dairy products, like cheese, cream, and whole milk. They can raise your blood cholesterol level.
    3. Cholesterol is found in foods from animals, such as egg yolks, liver, and high-fat meats and high-fat dairy products. Cholesterol in foods raises your blood cholesterol level.
    4. Trans fats are found in baked goods made with hydrogenated oil. Trans fats can also raise your cholesterol level.

Carbs give you calories and energy. But they also raise your blood glucose more than anything else you eat. Protein and fat give you calories and energy, too, but they don't raise your blood glucose. If you need to lose weight, though, using **portion power** for protein foods and fats will help you.

Most people I know are like me—they love carb foods. And many carb foods are healthy foods. Carbs provide good taste, pleasure, energy, vitamins, minerals, and fiber. Even though carbs raise blood glucose more than other foods, it's important for you to have some carbohydrates. For many reasons, then, "carbs count." If you can get the right balance between the amount of carbs you eat and your insulin or diabetes pills, that will help keep your blood glucose in your target range.

The first thing many people ask me is: "How many carbs can I eat?" For many people, having:

- 3 or 4 carb choices at each meal and
- 1 or 2 carb choices at snacks

is about right. Then round out your lunch or dinner with:

- 1 serving of meat, fish, or poultry, about 3 ounces
- Plenty of colorful veggies, such as green beans, broccoli, red peppers, or cabbage
- Healthy fats, like canola or olive oil, nuts, seeds, or avocado

Here is a meal that has 4 carb choices (the carb choices are in **bold print,** so you can see them):

- **3 small corn tortillas** (3 carb choices) with meat, salsa, lettuce, and chopped tomato
- **1/3 cup of rice** (1 carb choice)

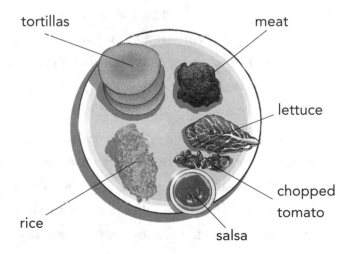

But what about portion sizes for carbs? **Portion power** with carbs helps keep your blood glucose in your target range. And by keeping your blood glucose levels in your target range, you can prevent or delay diabetes problems.

Take a look at the serving size guide below.

Carb Choice	Serving Size	Example (each has ~15 grams of carbs)
Bread	1 slice	1 small tortilla
Starchy side dishes		
rice or noodles, cooked	1/3 cup	1/3 cup spaghetti or rice
corn	1/2 cup	1/2 large ear of corn
Fruit	1/2 cup or 1 piece	1 small apple
Milk	1 cup (8 ounces)	1 small carton
Sweets	2-inch square	1 small piece of cake, unfrosted
	Amount to equal 15 grams of carbs	2 small cookies (check the food label)

Earlier I mentioned that my mom has diabetes. A few years ago, after Thanksgiving, she was diagnosed with type 2 diabetes. Mama was having severe back problems and wasn't able to be very active. But she and my dad were still enjoying the holidays with more food, which meant more calories. As a result, her weight went up to its highest point ever. As part of a routine checkup, her doctor checked her blood glucose level. Her blood glucose indicated she might have diabetes, so her doctor checked again a week later. Her blood glucose was still too high. Mama was scared when she was diagnosed with diabetes. She was scared because her sister had died from diabetes problems. But she was also surprised. She said she never thought she would have to worry about diabetes—even though diabetes ran in her family.

Her doctor signed her up for diabetes education classes at one of the local hospitals. While she was waiting to attend the classes and see a dietitian, she wanted me to be her dietitian! She wanted to get started right away. I told her it would be hard to be her daughter and her dietitian at the same time. She needed her own dietitian. But while she was waiting to see the dietitian, we got started. She and I talked about Rate Your Plate. After rating her own dinner plate, she decided she was eating way too many carbs. Mama loves carbs like I do—like mother like daughter, they always say. She also knew she and her doctor had agreed that she'd work on losing 15 pounds. We then talked about carb counting and trying for 3 carb choices at each meal and 1 carb choice for an evening snack.

Mama wanted her carb counting to be as simple as possible. She didn't want to be looking things up in a book all the time. Here's what we worked out for her to count as 1 carb choice:

1/2	cup of any starchy food, such as potatoes, cooked beans, peas, or corn
1/3	cup of cooked pasta or rice
1	small piece of fruit or 1/2 cup of fruit
1	cup of milk or yogurt
1/2	cup of low-fat ice cream or frozen yogurt
2	small cookies

1   handful (about 3/4 ounce) of pretzels, baked chips, or snack crackers

1   small dinner roll, tortilla, or muffin

1   piece of bread, 1 biscuit, 1/2 English muffin, 1/2 hamburger or hot dog bun, or 1/4 of a bakery bagel

1   cup of soup, such as chicken noodle, tomato, or split pea

1/2   cup of cooked cereal, such as oatmeal or grits

3/4   cup of dry ready-to-eat cereal, such as Cheerios

Any food that contains about 15 grams of total carbohydrate on the Nutrition Facts Label (see page 26 to learn more about reading food labels).

Mama thought the serving sizes seemed awfully small, especially that 1/4 bagel. Then we talked about having 3 carb choices at breakfast. Three carbs could be a 1/2 bagel (2 carb choices) and a 1/2 cup orange juice (1 carb choice) to drink with her medicine. That seemed more like something she could do. Today Mama skips the orange juice and drinks low-sodium vegetable juice to take her medicines. She likes saving that carb for fresh fruit or jam.

Next we did some meal planning for lunch and dinner. She decided on a sandwich on whole wheat bread (2 carb choices) and some baked chips (1 carb choice) for lunch. For dinner she wanted all 3 of her carb choices as spaghetti (about 1 cup, cooked).

For her bedtime snack, Mama said she would have a piece of fruit (1 carb choice), like a peach, apple, or orange. Or she might choose a glass of 1% milk for 1 carb. Or she might have a cup of light yogurt, like lemon or blackberry, for 1 carb. Or a couple of small cookies would be 1 carb.

"This isn't so hard," Mama said. "It's like I have a bank account of carbs for my meals and my evening snack. Then I spend the carbs in my bank account for the foods I love."

Then she thought about the rest of her meals. "But what about the rest of my meal?" Mama asked. "What about the meat and my salad with dressing?" I suggested she try for about 3 ounces of lean meat, poultry, or fish.

"I don't love meat the way I love carbs, but I'm not sure how much 3 ounces would be," Mama said. "And I need this to be simple. I don't have all day to be weighing and measuring my food. Besides, I thought you said carbs were what would raise my blood glucose."

"That's right, carbs are what raise blood glucose, but because you want to lose weight, you'll want to watch your portions of meats, too," I said.

"So **portion power** is coming into play with meats, too," Mama said. "How can I keep this simple?" We decided to look at a serving of 3 ounces of fish, poultry, or meat this way:

- a meat patty or serving the size of a mayonnaise jar lid
- a serving the size of the palm of your hand
- a serving the size of a deck of cards
- a serving the size of a checkbook

- a serving of three meatballs the size of ping pong balls or golf balls

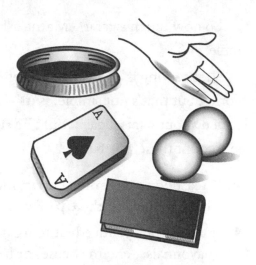

"Those would all fill about one-fourth of my plate, just like when I rate my plate," Mama said. "That makes sense to me. But what about tuna fish or cottage cheese—how do you count them?" she asked. We decided to count half of a 5- or 6-ounce can of water-packed tuna or 3/4 cup of low-fat cottage cheese the same as 3 ounces of meat.

"But what about regular cheese—how do I count it?" Mama asked.

"Mama," I said, "1 slice of cheese would be equal to 1 ounce of meat. Or a 1-inch cube of cheese, say, the size of 4 dice, would be equal to 1 ounce of meat. You know that a lot of cheeses are high in fat and cholesterol. Think about choosing fat-free or low-fat cheeses when you can. This will be good for your heart and blood cholesterol level."

"That reminds me that we haven't talked about fats yet, like margarine and oils," Mama said. "I know they say to eat less fat to lose weight."

"That's right, Mama," I said. "Fats have twice as many calories as carbs or protein. So choosing one or two fats at a meal or snack would be about the right amount."

"So how much is a fat?" Mama asked. "And keep it simple."

"A fat serving is about 5 grams of fat and about 45 calories, but that's not simple, is it?" I said. Mama and I decided about 4 fats a day would be right for her and that she'd count these as 1 fat:

- 1 teaspoon margarine, butter, mayonnaise, or oil. That's about the size of the **tip** of your thumb.
- 1 tablespoon reduced-fat margarine, reduced-fat mayonnaise, cream cheese, or half-and-half cream, the size of the **pad** of your thumb.
- 2 tablespoons reduced-fat salad dressing, reduced-fat cream cheese, or reduced-fat sour cream. Two tablespoons would be about half a ladle of dressing at a salad bar.

"How would you like some good news, Mama?" I asked.

"What's good about having diabetes?" she asked.

"The **good news** is that sometimes finding out you have diabetes is a wake-up call," I said. "People eat better, lose weight, get more active, start feeling better, and just enjoy life more. But the best news about diabetes is that you can prevent or delay diabetes problems like the problems Aunt Carla had."

"That is the best news I've had in a long time!" Mama said. "Is that all there is to eating with diabetes?"

"That's a good start, Mama," I said. "Plus just keep on making healthy food choices."

Then the time arrived for Mama's diabetes education

classes. I told Mama that she needed to tell her dietitian the way she likes to eat and then work together to design her own meal plan.

Your meal plan needs to fit your schedule, your likes and dislikes in foods, how active you are, when you like to eat, and where you go when you eat out. You and your dietitian will then design a meal plan that will fit the way you live and will include the foods you and your family like.

Luckily, a diabetes meal plan is good for the whole family. Making one dinner is hard, but making two—one for you and one for your family—just won't work. The foods you choose for taking care of your diabetes are the same foods that we all need to eat to stay healthy, whether we have prediabetes or diabetes or not. It's been great that Dad has been part of Mama's diabetes team. He's helping her count carbs. In fact, he's lost about 10 pounds by rating his plate and counting his carbs, too. And he's starting to walk some. Mama has been a good role model for him.

The first day of Mama's classes, a nurse educator talked to the group about diabetes in general, about checking blood glucose, and about things that affect blood glucose. Many family members, like me, were there to learn about diabetes care. They asked lots of questions and learned from each other.

Mama then worked with Marion, a dietitian and CDE. Marion started by talking about Carb Counting with Mama. Marion was pleased to learn that Mama had already started counting her carbs. Marion agreed that 3 carb choices at meals and 1 carb choice for a bedtime snack was a good starting point for her. Marion told Mama the next step was to start checking her blood glucose to see how this plan was working for her. For more on checking your blood glucose, see Chapter 7 (starting on page 57).

Next, Marion had Mama look at a food label. The Nutrition Facts label can help with meal planning. It can also help you make better food choices when you're shopping.

In the food label shown on the next page, let's go through the steps together to see how it can help you.

Steps in Using a Food Label

Step 1—Serving size. Look first at the serving size. All of the numbers in the Nutrition Facts box are based on this serving size. Is this the serving size you will be eating? How many servings are in the container or bag? In the sample label, one serving of macaroni and cheese equals 1 cup. If you ate the whole package, you would eat 2 cups. That doubles the calories and other nutrients.

Step 2—Calories. Now look at the calorie section of the label. It can help you with your weight. On this label, one serving of macaroni and cheese is 1 cup and 250 calories. If you eat 2 cups, it will be 500 calories. Eating too many calories will lead to weight gain.

Step 3—Total fat, saturated fat, trans fat, cholesterol, and sodium. Look at the grams of total fat, saturated fat, trans fat, and cholesterol. Eating too much of these fats may increase your risk of heart disease, some cancers, or high blood pressure. The same is true for sodium (salt).

1	Start Here ———	**Nutrition Facts**		
		Serving Size 1 cup (228g)		
		Servings Per Container 2		
		Amount Per Serving		
2	Check calories ———	**Calories** 250	**Calories from Fat** 110	
			% Daily Value**	
3	Limit these ——— nutrients	**Total Fat** 12g*	**18%**	
		Saturated Fat 3g	**15%**	
		Trans Fat 3g		
		Cholesterol 30mg	**10%**	
		Sodium 470mg	**20%**	
4	Review total ——— carbohydrates	**Total Carbohydrate** 31g	**10%**	
		Dietary Fiber 0g	**0%**	
		Sugars 5g		
		Protein 5g	**10%**	
5	Get enough ——— of these	Vitamin A 4% • Vitamin C 2%		
		Calcium 20% • Iron 4%		

*Amount in Cereal. One half cup of fat free milk contributes an additional 40 calories, 65mg sodium, 6g total carbohydrates (6g sugars), and 4g protein.
**Percent Daily Values are based on a 2,000 calorie diet. Your Daily Values may be higher or lower depending on your calorie needs.

	Calories:	2,000	2,500
Total Fat	Less than	65g	80g
Sat Fat	Less than	20g	25g
Cholesterol	Less than	300mg	300mg
Sodium	Less than	2,400mg	2,400mg
Potassium		3,500mg	3,500mg
Total Carbohydrate		300g	375g
Dietary Fiber		25g	30g

Calories per gram:
Fat 9 • Carbohydrate 4 • Protein 4

Experts suggest eating as little saturated fat, trans fat, cholesterol, and sodium as you can.

Step 4—Total carbohydrates. How many grams of carbohydrate are there in one serving? Mama said 31 grams, and she was right! If you eat two servings, it would be 62 grams, which is too high for most meals.

Divide total grams of carbohydrate by 15 to find out the number of carb choices. One serving of the macaroni and cheese would be 2 carb choices because 31 grams divided by 15 equals 2.

Step 5—Fiber, vitamins A and C, calcium, and iron. Most of us don't have enough dietary fiber, vitamins A and C, calcium, or iron in our meal plans. They are identified in the food label on page 27. Eating enough of these nutrients can improve your health and help reduce your risk of some diseases. For example, getting enough calcium may reduce the risk of brittle bones as we get older. That condition is called osteoporosis. Eating plenty of dietary fiber promotes healthy bowel function. Make an effort to choose fruits, vegetables, and grain products that contain dietary fiber.

You can use the Nutrition Facts label to compare products. Let's say you're shopping for canned soup. By looking at the Nutrition Facts label, you will be able to tell which brand is lower in calories, total fat, trans fat, cholesterol, and sodium.

You may be thinking that using the Nutrition Facts label will take more shopping time. That's true the first few times you use the label. But over time, you will find that it is a great tool to use for healthier shopping and eating.

Making Healthy Food Choices

Marion, the dietitian, and Mama then talked about making healthy food choices when planning meals. Marion suggested eating a wide variety of foods daily. Marion said this meant:

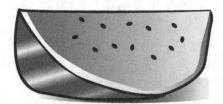

- Eating some fruit each day.
- Eating lots of vegetables that aren't starchy, such as tomatoes, cabbage, asparagus, cauliflower, green beans, broccoli, carrots, mushrooms, okra, leafy greens, and turnips.

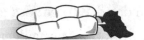

- Trying to eat different colored fruits and vegetables, such as dark green (collards or broccoli), orange (cantaloupe, apricots, or carrots), red (watermelon or tomatoes), blue (blueberries), and white (banana, cauliflower, or turnips). Some people call this "eating the rainbow." Research shows that eating colorful fruits and veggies also helps prevent cancer and heart disease.
- Choosing different kinds of starches, such as corn tortillas, black or pinto beans, hominy, whole-grain breakfast cereals and breads, and sweet potatoes.
- Eating high-fiber foods, like beans, whole-grain breads and cereals, and fruits and vegetables.
- Checking food labels for breakfast cereals that have at least 4 grams of fiber per serving.
- Looking for breads that have 2 to 3 grams of fiber per slice.
- Choosing dairy products that are low in fat. Nonfat (or skim) milk and 1% milk are the good choices. Light

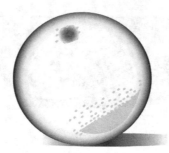

yogurts are also great when you want something sweet. Check the Nutrition Facts label for yogurts that are sweetened with a calorie-free sweetener.

Mama and Marion decided to choose only one or two changes for Mama to work on. Mama decided she wanted to eat more colorful fruits and vegetables. She thought it sounded like fun to eat the rainbow.

You may want to think about doing some of these things—one at a time—along with Rate Your Plate or Carb Counting. Read through the list of ideas above, and pick one action item you want to work on.

☞ This week, I'll work on _____

_____.

☞ The following week, I'll work on _____

_____.

Marion gave Mama a longer list of carb choices. That list is at the end of this book in Chapter 21, Diabetes Tools. If you decide to count your carbs, this longer list on page 190 may come in handy later on.

Glycemic Index

Mama heard about the **glycemic (gly-SEE-mik) index** on TV. The glycemic index is a number that tells you how much a carb food will raise blood glucose. A carb food may raise blood glucose a lot, a little, or somewhere in between.

Mama called and said, "I'm confused by this glycemic index. I thought all carbs raised blood glucose."

"You're right," I said. "All carbs do raise blood glucose, but some carbs raise blood glucose levels more than others. For example, corn flakes raise blood glucose more than oatmeal. For some people, using the glycemic index can help them keep their blood glucose on target."

"Well, what carbs raise blood glucose less?" Mama asked.

"The glycemic index for a food is not the same for everyone. The glycemic index of a food is also not the same for every meal. It depends on what else is in the meal, such as foods containing fiber or protein. It also depends on how well a food is cooked, like how long you cook your pasta. Research shows that you may have lower blood glucose levels after eating a meal if you choose low glycemic index foods, such as:

- dense and chewy breads rather than white bread
- breakfast cereals made with oats, barley, or bran. Oatmeal or all-bran cereals raise blood glucose less than cornflakes or toasted rice cereals.
- pasta more often than potatoes. Cooking pasta for shorter times, sometimes called "al dente," keeps blood glucose levels down more than soft, overcooked pasta.
- converted rice or long-grain rice. They raise blood

glucose a little less than short-grain rice.

- milk and yogurt
- plenty of non-starchy veggies, such as green beans or greens
- fruits, such as apples and oranges
- pinto, navy, lima, or kidney beans as well as chickpeas and lentils
- sweet potatoes. They raise blood glucose less than white potatoes.
- new potatoes. They raise blood glucose less than baked or mashed potatoes.

"It's best to choose the carbs you love so you feel satisfied. When you can, eat the carb foods that raise blood glucose less. Since you like oatmeal, Mama, having it a few times a week may help your blood glucose levels. Since you like pasta, have it instead of potatoes when it works into your meal.

"The glycemic index is just another tool that you can use to keep your blood glucose in your target range after meals."

Mama said, "So if I choose my favorite low-glycemic foods like beans and barley more often, it may help my blood glucose level."

"Yes, you've got it."

Using Meal Planning Tools

Rate Your Plate or Carb Counting works for most of my clients. Take Michael, for instance. He was 18 years old when I first started working with him. His doctor referred Michael to me because his blood fats and blood glucose were both too high. Michael didn't have diabetes, but he did have prediabetes. Prediabetes is the condition that comes before diabetes. It means that blood glucose levels are higher than normal but aren't high enough to be called diabetes. Like many people, Michael had prediabetes and didn't know it until he saw his doctor and had his blood glucose checked. People with prediabetes might get type 2 diabetes soon or later on.

Michael had a number of risks for diabetes:

- Diabetes runs in his family.
- He was very inactive.
- He had gained weight.

Michael had played football and used to work out at the school gym. Then he had an injury and couldn't play football anymore. He stopped going to the gym, and his weight went up. When he went to the doctor for his college physical, he found out he had prediabetes and high blood fats. Michael was shocked. He knew his grandparents had diabetes. And he knew about the problems that diabetes can bring. His grandmother had eye and kidney problems from her diabetes. And his grandfather had foot problems from his type 2 diabetes. But Michael was surprised about having prediabetes, because he was so young. After all, he was only 18 years old and just getting ready to go to college.

For Michael's visit with me, I asked him to bring a record of everything he ate and drank for 3 days. His record is on the next page.

Michael's Food Record

Breakfast	Large bowl of cereal with whole milk, 2–3 cups apple juice
Lunch	Large meatball sub, chips, large soda
Snack	Frozen waffle with peanut butter and lots of syrup, big glass of milk
Dinner	Barbequed ribs, potato salad, baked beans
Snack	Bag of microwave popcorn with a large soda

Michael said, "I tend to eat a good amount when I go out to eat. There's usually nothing left on my plate. I'm also crazy with sauces, catsup, and gravies. I put them on everything.

"I also like to eat fast food, like the meatball sub I had at lunch yesterday," Michael said. "I will sometimes super size my meal to get a bigger serving of fries and a larger drink."

Michael wanted to make changes to prevent getting type 2 diabetes and to lose weight for college. We talked about Rate Your Plate and Carb Counting. He decided he wanted to rate his plate. He also wanted to start going to the gym again.

He still wanted to eat out with his friends. We talked about picking lower-calorie choices when he was eating out. Michael decided he'd choose smaller portions and not super size his meals. He decided to drink diet soft drinks.

Michael and I reviewed the difference in calories and fat when he switched from a meatball sub to a turkey sub:

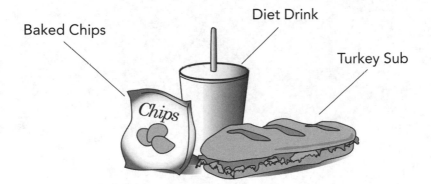

Baked Chips

Diet Drink

Turkey Sub

Chips

"Wow!" Michael said. "I never dreamed I could save 600 calories by switching from the meatball sub to the turkey sub and by choosing baked chips and a diet drink. That's a painless change I can make right away."

Michael did well. In 3 months, he had lost 10 pounds and was at the goal weight he had set for himself. And his blood glucose and cholesterol levels were back in the normal ranges.

Michael said, "I'm going to keep watching what I eat and being active. I really enjoy feeling and looking better. And I want to beat the odds and keep from getting type 2 diabetes."

—4—

Meal Planning and Shopping

We plan so many things in our lives. We make to-do lists to get things done. We make plans to see our friends on Friday night. We visit with our family over the weekend. We plan birthday parties for friends and family. We plan camping and fishing trips.

But many people I work with never plan meals. They spend a lot of time stopping at the grocery store to pick up something for dinner. Or they might pick up carry-out or fast food.

Planning your meals is a helpful tool whether you have diabetes or not. Meal planning helps in many ways. We can plan meals that:

- will include the foods we love
- follow our meal plan
- contain low-fat protein sources, such as lean chops, chicken breasts, fish, shellfish, and roasts

- include fruits and vegetables, with all the colors of the rainbow
- will save money and time!

So how does meal planning work? Here are the steps that many of my clients use for successful meal planning:

- Use a calendar or a form for each week. There's a form that you can use on page 196 in Chapter 21, Diabetes Tools. A sample of a completed form appears at the end of this chapter on page 42. Or you can use a calendar on your computer or phone.

- First fill in your schedule for the week. You may have a support group on Wednesday nights. Write that in. If you're having lunch with a friend on Monday, write that in. If you have a diabetes visit with your health care team on Thursday at 2:00 p.m., write that in. If you're having a friend over for a meal, write that in. And so on. In other words, write in all of your plans for the week.

- Next, plan your meals and snacks for each day, taking into account your schedule for the week. You may have quick breakfasts during the week, like ready-to-eat cereal with fresh fruit or an English muffin with a tablespoon of peanut butter and a banana. On Saturday, you may plan a breakfast that takes more time, like eggs and toast. On Sunday, you might eat a bagel with light cream cheese.

- Plan your lunches. Perhaps you want to use foods you can carry with you for lunch, like a turkey sandwich on whole-wheat pita bread, baked chips, raw veggies, and an apple. Peanut butter on graham crackers, baby carrots, an apple, and a small can of vegetable juice make for a fast lunch that is easy to put together. Or you may want to plan a main course salad for lunch one day. It might be a taco salad using leftover chicken and beans with salad greens and other veggies. Top it with salsa or salsa mixed with low-fat French dressing. Have fat-free tortilla chips on the side. If you plan to buy lunch, write that on your calendar.

- It's a good idea to plan foods for your snacks so you'll have foods you enjoy and that match your meal plan. Your snack could be low-fat or fat-free cheese with a pear, pretzels, graham crackers, or light yogurt.

- Now to dinners. If you have a support group meeting at night, you may want to purchase a main course frozen dinner that can be prepared quickly. Add a vegetable or salad and a whole-grain roll for a complete meal. Write that on your calendar. Other nights you may want to make a simple and fast meal of a baked potato topped with low-fat canned chili or a baked potato topped with cottage cheese and salsa. All you need to go with these meals is frozen broccoli or some other frozen vegetable you like or maybe a salad. Think about the bags of prewashed salad greens, or purchase greens and veggies from a salad bar to save time.

- Plan for leftovers. When you grill chicken and vegetables, make extras for lunch or another night later on. If you have a casserole, make two and freeze one. It will taste great in a month.

- Think about trying a new recipe every week or so. This keeps your meals interesting. This can also keep you from feeling deprived or bored with your meals. Check out all the many diabetes cookbooks that provide the amount of carbs, calories, and fat for each serving. (There are many cookbooks published by the ADA that can be purchased at www.shopdiabetes.org or call 1-800-232-6733.)

- After you have your weekly menu planned, it's time to make your shopping list. Take into account what you already have on hand. Check your cupboards and freezer to see what you might want to use this week. Maybe use up the pork roast or the chicken breasts that are in the freezer? What about the pasta in the cupboard or the canned tuna? Now make your shopping list. There's a shopping list in Chapter 21, Diabetes Tools, starting on page 198. It may be helpful. Or just make your own list on a piece of paper. You can also keep your shopping list on your computer or phone.

  Your shopping will go more quickly if you make your list match the layout of your store—fresh fruits and vegetables, then breads, fresh meat and poultry, dairy products, and so on. Write down the items you need to buy for the week. You might need fresh or frozen vegetables, fruit, milk, yogurt, bread, frozen dinners, chicken breasts, deli meats, low-fat cheese, and snack foods.

- If you like, you can use the bottom of the My Meal Plan form on page 196 in Chapter 21, Diabetes Tools, to keep track of your activities for the week. Writing down your biking or whatever you like to do makes you feel good about yourself. It also helps to keep you moving!

- As you run out of food items over the week, keep a running list of items you need to pick up. This list might include mustard, canned soups, chicken broth, canned tomatoes, rice, or tuna fish.

- When you do your shopping, you'll know exactly what you need to buy for the week. You'll be able go through the store more quickly.

- To save money, check weekly store sales and coupons. If you need turkey for your lunches, but ham is on sale, switch to the ham. If you have a coupon for yogurt, and yogurt is on your list, use the coupon. However, coupons for unhealthy foods or items you may not use aren't good buys.

- If you rely on your list, you'll save money in another way. You'll only buy what you will use. No more rotting fruits and vegetables that you have to throw away!

Taking the time to make a menu and a shopping list will save you time in the long run. You'll already know what you're eating when you get home late and need to make a quick dinner. Not only will your menus match your diabetes meal plan, they will also match your schedule for the week.

My Meal Plan
Date: May 7 to May 13

	Sunday	Monday	Tuesday
Breakfast	1/2 whole-grain bagel 1% milk 1 small apple	Raisin bran cereal 1% milk 1 small apple	Oatmeal 1% milk 1 slice toast
Snack	Small orange	Pretzels	6-ounce container light yogurt
Lunch	Baked chicken Mashed potatoes Green beans	Noon—lunch at Jane's house	Ham sandwich Leftover slaw Baked chips
Snack	3 cups low-fat popcorn	17 small grapes	1/2 cup light fruit cocktail
Dinner	Chicken sandwich Carrot sticks Baked chips	1 cup chili with beans 1 square cornbread Slaw	Leftover baked chicken 1 cup canned corn Frozen spinach
Snack	1/2 cup pudding	1/2 cup light ice cream	1/2 cup pineapple
Activity Today	Walked 1 hour at the zoo	Got off bus and walked 5 extra blocks	Walked to post office, 30 minutes

Wednesday	Thursday	Friday	Saturday
English muffin Peanut butter Small banana	Leftover oatmeal 1 slice whole-wheat toast 2 tablespoons raisins	English muffin 1 slice cheese 1/2 cup applesauce	Scrambled eggs 1 slice whole-wheat toast 1/2 grapefruit
3 graham crackers	Peach	2 breadsticks	1/2 cup Cheerios
1 can chicken noodle soup Crackers Pear	1 cup leftover chili with beans Crackers Carrot sticks	Frozen dinner Whole-wheat roll	2 slices cheese Toast Baked chips Celery sticks
6 ounce container light yogurt	2 pm—see Dr. Wood Apple	6 crackers	Fudgesicle
7:30 pm—support group Frozen dinner Frozen mixed veggies Dinner roll	Tuna fish salad Whole-wheat pita bread Baked chips Sliced tomatoes	7 pm—Robert over for dinner Pork chops Baked potato Salad Fresh mixed fruit	Grilled sirloin Rice Salad Green beans Watermelon
Orange	2 small cookies	1/2 cup light yogurt	3 cups popcorn at the movie
None	Worked out at the gym after seeing Dr. Wood, 1 hour	Ran errands and walked at lunch, 30 minutes	Walked 30 minutes while shopping at the mall

—5—

Tips for Eating Out with Diabetes

I'm old enough to remember when eating out was something special. It was someone's birthday, or it was when Aunt Betty came to visit.

Eating away from home isn't anything special anymore. A few of my clients eat out for all their meals. Others eat out 6 to 10 times a week. What's the problem with eating out? Here's my short list:

- Even though we eat out a lot, many of us still think it's a special treat and eat more than usual.
- To make things taste great and keep us coming back, chefs use more fat and sauces than we do at home. More fat means more calories.
- Portions of foods served in restaurants are getting bigger and bigger.
- Fast-food places try to make us think it's a better deal to "super size" our meal, and then we overeat.
- Fruits and vegetables are hard to find when we eat out.

- Desserts are sometimes big enough to serve four people!

Everyone loves to eat out. It's a way of life. It's how we get to see our friends and family. How often do we say, "Let's get together for lunch!"?

So let's tackle eating out step-by-step.

Top Tips for Eating Away from Home

1. Try to eat out no more than three times a week. You'll save calories and money.

2. Know your meal plan, or write it down. How many carbs do you plan to eat?

3. Plan ahead. Think about what you'll order and how much you'll eat.

4. Call or check online if you're unsure of the menu. If you're not sure that you'll find the type of foods you want to order, go someplace else.

5. Work with your server. Here are some things you may want to ask:

   ○ How is the fish cooked? Is it grilled or fried?

   ○ Is there a sauce? Think about all the times you've been surprised by a sauce not mentioned on the menu. Ask for the sauce on the side.

   ○ Can you get a baked potato instead of fries?

   ○ Can you get the baked potato toppings, such as butter or sour cream, on the side?

   ○ Can you get salad dressings on the side?

   ○ If you made it clear you wanted your salad dressing

or the sauce on the side, and your plate arrives with your food swimming in sauce, send it back!

6. When your food arrives, compare it to your goals for the meal. How many carbs are in the rice? If there are two chicken breasts or two chops, think about taking one of them home for tomorrow's lunch, along with the extra rice.

7. Add sauces and salad dressings one of two ways:

   ○ Dip the tines of your fork into the sauce or dressing. Then spear a piece of meat or lettuce for a little sauce or dressing with each bite.

   ○ Add 1 teaspoon of dressing or sauce at a time. When you've eaten that, add another teaspoon.

   You'll eat less salad dressing or sauce using either of these methods.

8. At a fast-food place, ask them to leave off the mayo or sauces on sandwiches, and ask for a packet of mustard, catsup, or barbeque sauce. You'll eat fewer calories and less fat.

9. Stick with grilled, broiled, or baked fish, poultry, and meat.

10. Remove the skin from poultry. Trim fat off meats.

11. Order the smallest size of meat, such as a 4-ounce filet rather than a 12-ounce piece of prime rib. Besides having **portion power**, the filet will be lower in fat and calories.

12. Split an entrée with a family member or friend. You'll eat less and save money, too. Sometimes there will be a charge for splitting an entrée. You'll still come out ahead

two ways. You'll save the cost of the second entrée and also save on the extra calories, carbs, and fat.

13. Order two appetizers instead of a main course.

14. Don't forget about the bread basket or the tortilla basket. Can you eat just one piece of bread and count it as one of your carb choices? Or about 15 tortilla chips? Will this carb choice fit into the rest of the meal you've ordered? If not, move the basket away from you, or ask your server to take it away.

15. Use small amounts of fats like oil and butter. Or don't add extra. The chef has already added more than you or I can even guess.

16. If you want to Rate Your Plate, check the size of the plate when you eat out. Sometimes the plates are more like platters. Check the amount of food, and ask for a box to take any extra food home for a later meal. Studies show that the more we're served, the more we eat.

17. Split sweets and treats with a friend or family members. Order one dessert and four spoons!

This is a long list of tips for eating away from home. Pick one tip to work on. When you have mastered it, pick one or two more to try.

☞ When I eat out this week, I'll _____

_____

☞ When I eat out next week, I'll _____

_____.

—6—

What to Eat When You're Sick

Like everyone else, people with diabetes get sick. They get colds, the flu, or an upset stomach. When you get sick, take extra care of yourself to keep your blood glucose levels in your target range.

Work with your health care team to design your sick day plan. Until you do, here are some tips you can use for sick days.

Tips for Sick Days

- Check your blood glucose every 4 hours, and write down the results.
- Check your temperature when you check your blood glucose.
- Drink plenty of fluids, about 8 ounces at a time. If your temperature is over 99 degrees, drink some fluids hourly.
- Check for ketones, if you take insulin and your blood

glucose levels are over 300. (See page 71 for more on ketones.)

- Take your diabetes medicines. An illness can make your blood glucose go up.

  - Take your usual diabetes pills, except for the pills you take only when you eat.
  - If you use insulin, take your usual dose. If your blood glucose level is high, check with your health care team. You may need extra insulin until you're feeling better.

- Eat your usual amount of carbohydrates in your meal plan.

  - If you have an upset stomach or are vomiting, try to take enough fluids that contain carbs to equal the carbohydrates in your meal plan. Space the fluids out over the day. Taking a few sips every 15 minutes may help keep fluids down. Often sodas, such as ginger ale, help with nausea, and they contain carbohydrates.
  - If you have a sore throat, try soft foods, such as yogurt or a baked potato, to get your carbohydrates in a way that won't hurt your throat.

Liquid and Soft Sick Day Foods

The foods listed on the next page each have about 15 grams of carbohydrate and can be used in your meal plan when you are sick with a cold, flu, or upset stomach or when you have dental work. The amount of food can be doubled or tripled if you need more carbohydrates for your meal plan.

15-Gram Carb Foods	Amount
Regular (not diet) soft drink	1/2 cup
Juices	1/2 cup
Sports drinks	1 cup
Milk	1 cup
Yogurt, plain or light	1 cup
Chocolate milk	1/2 cup
Milk shake	1/2 cup
Regular (not sugar-free) Jell-O	1/2 cup
Fruit cup	1/2 cup
Applesauce	1/2 cup
Banana	1 small
Cooked cereal	1/2 cup
Mashed potatoes	1/2 cup
Rice	1/3 cup
Cream or tomato soup (made with water)	1 cup
Cream or tomato soup (made with milk)	1/2 cup
Chicken noodle or chicken rice soup	1 cup
Crackers	6–8
Toast	1 slice
Pudding, regular	1/4 cup
Pudding, no-sugar-added	1/2 cup
Ice cream	1/2 cup
Frozen yogurt	1/2 cup
Sherbet or sorbet	1/4 cup
Fruit juice bars, frozen	1 bar
Jam or jelly	1 Tbsp
Honey	1 Tbsp
Sugar	1 Tbsp

Talk with your health care team about when to call if you're sick. Write down the phone numbers that you would call during the day and at night.

☞ Daytime telephone number: _____

☞ Evening telephone number: _____

In the meantime, here are some ideas for when to call.

When to Call Your Health Care Team

Call right away if you are:

- having blood glucose levels over 300
- vomiting or having diarrhea for more than 1 day
- running a high fever for more than 1 day. A high fever is over 101 degrees.
- sick for more than 2 days
- unable to eat for more than 1 day

When you call your health care provider, be ready to give this information:

☞ How long you've been sick: _____

☞ Your blood glucose levels: _____

☞ Your temperature: _____

☞ Medicines you're taking: _____

☞ How much you've been able to eat and drink:

_____

☞ Your symptoms: _____

☞ Your pharmacist's phone number: _____

☞ Contact information for a pharmacy that is open all
  night and on weekends: _____

After talking with your health care team about your own
plan for when you're sick, write below the reasons your
health care team says you need to call.

Reasons to Call My Diabetes Health Care Team

☞ _____

☞ _____

☞ _____

☞ _____

☞ _____

☞ _____

☞ _____

Feeling Bad: A Real Life Story

Robert had a bad cough, sore throat, and runny nose that kept getting worse. His blood glucose levels were getting higher and higher, too. He went to the drugstore and bought some cough syrup and some cold pills. After 2 days of not getting better and running a fever, he called his health care team.

Robert reported:

- 3 days of being sick
- blood glucose levels of 200 in the mornings and in the 300s during the day
- a temperature of 100
- taking his diabetes, blood pressure, and cholesterol medicines plus cough syrup and cold pills
- eating soft foods and liquids to get all the carbs in his meal plan
- a very sore throat, bad cough, runny nose, and not sleeping

Robert was given an appointment for that afternoon. Robert brought along his logbook of blood glucose readings and of the medicines he had been taking. His team checked his blood pressure, temperature, and blood glucose and listened to his heart and his breathing. Robert had bronchitis (brong-KI-tis) and needed an antibiotic. The doctor raised his insulin dose to get his blood glucose levels down. He also told Robert to keep eating all the carbs in his meal plan and to drink plenty of fluids. His team said to call if he didn't feel better in a day or so. He was also to call if his blood glucose levels didn't drop after the added insulin.

After 10 days, Robert was back to his old self. The cough was gone, his breathing was normal, and he was hungry and ate his full meal plan. Robert's team asked him to continue checking his blood glucose levels more often for another few days after he went back to his regular dose of insulin.

—7—

Checking Your Blood Glucose

Keeping your blood glucose close to your target range is your best route for good health. You'll feel better, too. Checking your blood glucose is the only way to know how your blood glucose is doing. Your doctor will tell you how often or if you need to check your blood glucose.

Some people with diabetes think they can guess when their blood glucose is high or low. But studies show they're wrong most of the time when they just guess.

Research shows that keeping your blood glucose close to your target range can lower your risk for diabetes problems, also called complications. You can keep track of your blood glucose levels in two ways:

1. **Use a meter to check your blood glucose.** This gives you a snapshot of your blood glucose level at that moment. Your diabetes team will teach you how to check.

2. **Ask your doctor or nurse to order an A1C or eAG.**
The A1C (A-one-see) or eAG (estimated average glucose)
check is the blood glucose check with a memory. It tells
you your average estimated blood glucose level over the
past 2 to 3 months. The eAG expresses your A1C in the
same units as your glucose meter.

Using a Blood Glucose Meter

By using your results from both of these checks, you and your
diabetes team will know how your diabetes plan is working.
These checks will also help you and your diabetes team know
when to make changes in your diabetes plan.

At Mama's second diabetes
education class, a nurse gave her a
meter and showed her how to check
her blood glucose. The nurse
explained to Mama that blood
glucose levels go up and down all day
long. The nurse said, "Checking
blood glucose any time and any
place, and keeping track of the
results, will help you know what's going on with your blood
glucose. You'll see what food, exercise, stress, and medicine
do to your blood glucose levels."

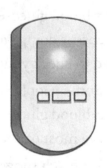

Sometimes it's tricky to learn how to use a meter. When
Mama got home from her class, she tried to check her blood
glucose. Her meter kept giving her an error message, so she

knew something wasn't right. She called me, but I wasn't at home. She called the diabetes educator, but she had left for the day. She then called her pharmacist, who had sold her the strips she needed for her meter. The pharmacist went through the steps for her meter with Mama. Always remember that you have many members on your diabetes team—your doctor, dietitian, nurse, pharmacist, family, and friends. Don't be afraid to ask them to help when you have a problem. Also, most meter companies have toll-free customer service numbers you can call for help. Some meters come with a video that shows how to use your meter.

Mama now checks her blood glucose without any problems. She likes seeing how the foods she eats affect her blood glucose. She also likes seeing how much walking or yard work lowers her blood glucose levels.

It's a good idea to have your nurse or dietitian watch as you check your blood glucose using your meter. Then you'll know your meter is giving you the right blood glucose readings.

How Often Do I Check My Blood Glucose?

Many people check their blood glucose several times a day—before or after meals and before bedtime. Others check less often. Talk with your diabetes team about when and how often to check your blood glucose. Then write down the times to check in your logbook or here, as a reminder:

☞ I need to check my blood glucose at least _____ times a day.

☞ I need to check my blood glucose:

- [ ] When I get up in the morning
- [ ] 2 hours after meals
- [ ] 2 hours after snacks
- [ ] Before going to bed

In the beginning, Mama's doctor wanted her to check her blood glucose twice a day and at different times of the day. He also asked Mama to write down her blood glucose results in a logbook he gave her.

BLOOD SUGAR RECORD

	BREAKFAST		LUNCH		DINNER		BEDTIME	
	before	after	before	after	before	after	before	after
MON.								
TUE.								
WED.								
THU.								
FRI.								
SAT.								
SUN.								

If you need a logbook, look in Chapter 21, Diabetes Tools, on page 194. There's a log you can copy into a notebook, or you can copy it on a copy machine. You can also keep track of your blood glucose results on your computer or phone.

One morning, Mama checked her blood glucose before she had anything to eat or drink. This is called fasting blood glucose, since she hadn't eaten or drunk anything since the night before. That same day, Mama checked her blood glucose 2 hours after she started to eat breakfast. The next day, she checked her blood glucose two different times: 2 hours after she started to eat lunch and 2 hours after she started to eat her bedtime snack. The next day, she checked her blood glucose first thing in the morning and 2 hours after she started to eat dinner.

At her next doctor visit, Dr. Wood reviewed Mama's blood glucose logbook with her. He said her diabetes plan seemed to be working because her blood glucose levels were within her target range most of the time. Mama's doctor then said she only needed to check her blood glucose a few times a week. But Mama thinks that checking her blood glucose more often and getting feedback help her keep her blood glucose on track.

The A1C or eAG Check

To be sure her diabetes plan was on target, Mama's doctor also checked her A1C, the blood check with a memory, to find out how her average blood glucose had been for the last 2 to 3 months.

"Mrs. Mathews, you're doing a great job," said Dr. Wood. "And your diabetes plan is working well. Your A1C is down almost a point. That's very good. Your hard work is paying off. The lower your A1C is, the lower your chances are of having any diabetes problems. Let's continue to work toward your A1C target of 6."

If your A1C is	Then your estimated average glucose (eAG) is
6	126
7	154
8	183
9	212
10	240
11	269
12	298

Look at the table above and find your last A1C result in the left column. Then look across to learn your average blood glucose for the past 2 to 3 months. If you don't know your A1C, talk with your doctor or nurse to find out your A1C result.

The A1C checks include all the highs and lows and tell you what your average blood glucose has been over the last 2 to 3 months. You can't get this information from your checks with your blood glucose meter. Your A1C result gives you the big picture on how your treatment plan is working. And it's worth repeating that the lower your A1C is, the lower your chances are of getting any long-term diabetes problems.

The American Diabetes Association recommends getting your A1C checked at least every 6 months and more often if you're not meeting your blood glucose goals. The higher your A1C number, the higher your risk for diabetes problems. If your A1C number is 7 or higher, you may need a change in your diabetes plan to get it lower. Talk with your doctor or health care team.

Dr. Wood said the A1C goal for my mom is 6. Talk with your doctor about your A1C goal and write it here:

☞ My target for the A1C check is _____.

☞ My last A1C result was _____.

The American Diabetes Association A1C goal is below 7 for most people with diabetes.

—8—

Keeping Your Blood Glucose in Your Target Range

Do you know your blood glucose goals? If you don't, ask your diabetes health care team what yours are. Keeping blood glucose in your target range helps prevent diabetes problems later on, and you'll feel better every day, too. Dr. Wood is following the American Diabetes Association guidelines for his patients. These guidelines are listed below. Your doctor and diabetes team may decide on a different target range for you.

Talk with your diabetes team, and set your target blood glucose range. Then fill in the blanks below:

☞ My blood glucose target before meals and when I wake up is _____ to _____.
(ADA goal is an average of 70 to 130.)

☞ My blood glucose target 2 hours after starting to eat a meal is below _____.
(ADA goal is below 180.)

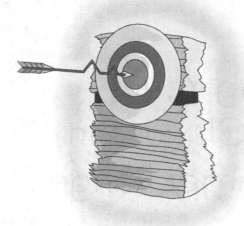

Checking your blood glucose at different times on different days gives you and your diabetes team the big picture of how your diabetes care plan is working. Write down the results, and use them to see how food, activity, and stress affect your blood glucose and to look for patterns. Patterns are similar blood glucose results over and over again. If your blood glucose is always high after breakfast or after dinner, talk with your diabetes team about making changes to bring it down.

—9—

What Makes Your Blood Glucose Go Up or Down?

Blood glucose levels rise and fall all day long, every day, for everyone. Your daily checks with your blood glucose meter give you a snapshot of your blood glucose at that moment.

Sometimes your blood glucose checks will show numbers out of your target range. When this happens to my mom, she says, "I don't like it!" Sometimes you know why your blood glucose is lower or higher than your target. Other times, you may not be able to figure it out. Think of blood glucose numbers as clues to what's going on. Take a close look at your blood glucose logbook to see if your blood glucose levels are too high or too low several days in a row at about the same time. This is called a pattern. If the same thing keeps happening over and over again, it might be time to change your diabetes plan. Talk with your diabetes team when you see this happening.

One key to taking care of your diabetes is learning why your blood glucose levels go up and down. If you know the reasons, you can take steps to keep your blood glucose in your target range.

Nathan, one of my clients, used to get high blood glucose after dinner. He said he would get home from work, tired and hungry, and nibble while he was making his dinner. Then he would eat his dinner. When he checked his blood glucose 2 hours after starting to eat dinner, his blood glucose would be 250 to 300.

Nathan decided he would make extra dinners on the weekend and freeze them. He also bought a supply of frozen dinners to have on hand. "All I have to do is heat something up when I get home," said Nathan. "I also keep fresh veggies handy in case I need a snack before dinner, since they don't raise my blood glucose."

Mama found out her blood glucose was higher when she skipped her walks. She also found out it went down when she did extra yard work, like raking leaves or pulling weeds. For more on exercise and diabetes, see Chapter 10 on page 77.

Nathan takes insulin and diabetes pills for his type 2 diabetes. His blood glucose goes up if he forgets to take his diabetes pills. It drops too low when Nathan eats his meals late.

Mama found out that there are many things that can make her blood glucose go up. She was having a bad time with pain in her back. She wasn't able to enjoy her walks. Dr. Wood suggested a new medicine for her back. He warned Mama that the medicine would make her blood glucose go up. Wow, was she surprised when it hit almost 300! Luckily, her blood glucose came down over time—and her back was much better. Now she can enjoy her walks again.

Mama's blood glucose went up for a few reasons. What are they?

- If you guessed her blood glucose went up from being less active, you're right.
- If you guessed her blood glucose went up from the side effects of the new medicine, you're right.
- If you guessed her blood glucose went up from the pain and stress on her body, you're right.

Mama learned that high blood glucose levels can result from more than one thing at the same time.

My cousin Pam has diabetes. Last year, Pam called me because her blood glucose was 285. She also said she was sick with the flu. I told her that being sick raises blood glucose. This year, Pam got a flu shot. To learn more about flu shots, see page 90.

Stress will also raise blood glucose. Like many people, Pam has stress at her job. Pam is trying to learn to let go of some things at work that are stressful for her. To learn more about stress and diabetes, see Chapter 15 on page 133.

So the main things that affect your blood glucose are:

- food
- amount of activity
- medicines
- illness
- stress

When your blood glucose is out of your target range, think about the meals and snacks you've eaten or have not eaten. Think about how active you've been. Think about how good or bad you feel. Are you coming down with something? Are you extra stressed or worried about work or something at home? These questions will help solve your blood glucose puzzle.

If Your Blood Glucose Is Too High

If your blood glucose is too high, you may:

- be more thirsty than usual
- urinate more often
- have dry or itchy skin
- have more infections
- have cuts or sores that heal more slowly
- feel sleepy
- have blurred vision

If your blood glucose is high, ask yourself these questions to figure out the reasons:

- Did I eat my meal or snack on time?
- Did I have a bigger-than-usual meal?
- Did I have a bigger-than-usual snack?
- Did I take my diabetes medicine earlier or later than usual?
- Did I take fewer pills or less insulin than my usual dose?

- Did I forget to take my pills or insulin?
- Did I take other medicines that may have made my blood glucose go up?
- Do I need a higher dose of pills or insulin?
- Do I feel like I'm getting a cold?
- Is my arthritis acting up?
- Was it the minor surgery?
- Was it the dental checkup?
- Am I worried about something?
- How about hormone levels? (For more on women's issues related to diabetes, see Chapter 17 on page 149.)

What Can I Do When My Blood Glucose Is High?

If your blood glucose is too high much of the time, work with your health care team to make changes to your meal plan, activity level, or diabetes medicines. You have the power to make the changes that will work for you.

Eating regular meals—but not overeating—can help. Exercising most days and taking your diabetes medicines as directed can also help prevent high blood glucose.

Exercise can lower your blood glucose. But if your blood glucose is higher than 300 and you take insulin, your health care provider may want you to check your blood or urine for ketones. Ketones are waste products made by your body when your blood glucose is high. Too many ketones can make you very sick. At your next diabetes visit, ask your provider whether you should exercise when your blood glucose is very high.

If Your Blood Glucose Is Too Low

Nathan started to feel shaky and weak. He checked his blood glucose—it was only 60! That's too low. He drank half a cup of juice, checked his blood glucose again after 15 minutes, and found that his blood glucose level had risen to 75. Nathan didn't know why his blood glucose had gone low. He asked himself these questions:

- Did I eat enough at my last meal?
- Did I eat earlier than usual?
- Did I skip any meals or snacks today?
- Did I eat enough carbohydrate foods?
- Did I have alcoholic drinks without eating? (For more on alcohol and diabetes, see page 153 in Chapter 18.)
- Was I more active than usual today?
- Did I take more diabetes pills or insulin than usual?
- Do I need to reduce the number of pills or the amount of insulin I take?

If your blood glucose level goes too low, you can use these same questions to try to find out what happened.

Low blood glucose is also called hypoglycemia (HY-poh-gly-SEE-mee-uh), when your blood glucose level drops below 70. People with type 2 diabetes who use meal planning and exercise don't normally get hypoglycemia.

When your blood glucose is this low, you may feel

- anxious
- confused
- dizzy
- grumpy
- hungry
- nervous
- shaky
- sweaty

What Can I Do When My Blood Glucose Is Too Low?

If you have these feelings and think your blood glucose is too low, use your meter to check your blood glucose level. If you find that your blood glucose is below 70, follow the 15-15 rule.

The 15-15 Rule

The 15-15 rule reminds you to

- eat 15 grams of carbohydrate
- wait 15 minutes
- check your blood glucose again

If your blood glucose is still below 70, eat another 15 grams of carbohydrate. You can get about 15 grams of carbohydrate from these **quick-fix foods and drinks**:

- 2 to 5 glucose tablets
- 1 serving of glucose gel (the amount that gives you 15 grams of carbohydrate—see the label on the package)
- 1/2 cup (4 ounces) fruit juice
- 1 cup (8 ounces) of milk
- 1/2 cup (4 ounces) of regular (not diet) soft drink
- 5 to 6 pieces of hard candy
- 1 tablespoon of sugar or honey

   (If you take a medication called an alpha-glucosidase inhibitor, only glucose tablets or gel can be used to treat lows.)

After 15 minutes, check your blood glucose again. If it's still below 70, have another 15 grams of a quick-fix food or drink. Repeat these steps until your blood glucose is above 70. Now eat a meal or snack to keep your blood glucose level where it needs to be.

If your blood glucose is too low too often, you need a change in your meal plan, your activity, or your diabetes medicines. Keep track of any low blood glucose levels in your logbook, and note the reasons, such as skipping a meal.

Always talk with your diabetes team about blood glucose levels that are too low or too high. Also, talk with your diabetes team about patterns you see in your logbook. You can work with your team to make a change in your diabetes plan.

Now you know that the major factors that can affect your blood glucose are:

- food
- exercise
- diabetes medicines
- side effects from other medicines
- being sick
- being stressed
- timing—the times you eat, exercise, and take your diabetes medicines

There are a lot of things that can affect your blood glucose. But checking your blood glucose will help you figure out what's going on. You'll see what food, exercise, stress, and medicines do to your blood glucose levels. You can learn how to use your blood glucose numbers to make changes in your diabetes plan.

Robert Says...

Robert says it takes time and effort to learn about what's going on with your blood glucose levels. He's learned that blood glucose levels go up for other reasons besides what you eat. Being sick, stressed, or tired can affect blood glucose. You need to know what's going on with your body.

—10—

Get Up and Get Going

Living an active life is a great way to take care of type 2 diabetes. It's also a great way to delay or prevent type 2 diabetes if you have prediabetes.

You don't have to spend hours working out in a gym to look and feel better! Just 30 minutes most days of the week will do it. You can even split it into two or three parts. Try a 10-minute walk after every meal. Or think of ways to build extra activity into your day. You don't have to go to a gym unless you want to. Just walk, mop the floor, wash the car, weed the garden, clean the house, or ride your bike. How about dancing? That's fun. Or go swimming. There are many fun things to do to get in motion. The choice is yours.

The American Diabetes Association recommends at least 150 minutes of moderate-intensity aerobic exercise per week. Spread this 150 minutes over at least 3 days, with no more than 2 days between exercise.

Exercise helps with prediabetes and type 2 diabetes. Exercise also helps in a lot of other ways. It can:

- relieve stress and promote calmness
- lower your blood glucose, blood pressure, and blood cholesterol levels
- use up extra glucose in your blood
- help your own insulin work better
- make your heart, muscles, and bones strong
- improve your blood flow
- tone your muscles
- help you lower your weight and lose inches off your waistline
- keep your body and your joints limber
- burn calories and increase endurance

So now you know that being active helps you lower your blood glucose, blood fats (cholesterol), and blood pressure. It also helps with weight loss. So what are you waiting for? Motion is the potion!

If you haven't been active for a while, check with your health care team first. You may need a checkup before you start being more active.

Here are a few ways to get in motion:

- Walk rather than driving your car or taking the bus.
- Take the stairs.
- Join an exercise group in your area.
- Start a walking group at work or in your neighborhood.

- Do the exercises on TV every morning at home, or record them for later. Exercise videos are ready when you are, too.
- Take a dance class.
- Walk at the mall.
- Walk around while talking on the phone.
- When shopping, take the faraway parking spot and walk to the store.
- Carry groceries to your car rather than driving to pick them up.
- Carry things in two trips instead of one.
- Walk to the mailbox or post office.
- Walk the dog after dinner.
- Play with the kids.
- Walk to the drugstore instead of driving or taking the bus.

Pick one thing from the list above to try.

☞ This week, I'll_____.

☞ Next week, I may try _____.

☞ Other things I am thinking of doing are _____
_____.

Mama loves to walk. She walks in her neighborhood, and sometimes her neighbors join in and they visit and talk. She tries to walk 30 minutes almost every day, but sometimes her back is acting up. Then she may walk 5 to 10 minutes several times a day.

When Mama's back is really giving her problems or it's raining, she may do armchair exercises. Her exercise therapist told her about armchair exercise videos she could borrow from the library or buy. Mama likes the seated exercises she does along with the video because she feels more flexible and limber after doing them. If you're interested in armchair exercises, talk with your diabetes health care team to see if seated exercises might be right for you. For more on armchair videos, check with your local library or go online.

Michael told me he wanted to be more active, but he didn't know what to do, since he couldn't play football anymore. I asked Michael to come up with a list of ideas of things he might want to do. Here's Michael's list:

- Go to the gym 2 days a week.
- Play softball with his friends.
- Walk and jog 2 days a week.

Michael decided to start by walking three times a week. When the weather is bad, he will go to the gym. Michael hopes to start strength training next month.

Get Ready to Be More Active

Take the first step toward making a plan to be more active. Talk with your diabetes team about what kinds of activities you think you would like to do.

You might do something that keeps your heart strong and uses up extra blood glucose and calories, like swimming, walking, or dancing. You also might do gentle stretching or strength training to keep your joints loose and your muscles strong.

If you have diabetes problems, talk with your diabetes team to find out which exercise choices are safe for you.

Get Set

When you've built up to longer and more active workouts, here are a few things to keep in mind:

- Ask your diabetes team about when to check your blood glucose. In general, check your blood glucose before you exercise. If it's below 100, have a carb snack that is about 15 grams carbohydrate. This might be a piece of fruit or a handful of pretzels before you start.
- Start slowly to warm up. Stretch your muscles. At the end, slow down to cool off before you stop.
- Stretch again to finish up.
- Attach your medical ID to your shoes or clothing, and carry a wallet-sized medical ID card, too.
- Carry a carb food with you. Then you'll be ready to treat low blood glucose if it happens. Glucose tablets, sugar packets, or small boxes of raisins are easy to carry.
- Drink plenty of water before, during, and after exercise.

Go for It: Making a Plan and Getting Started

Making a plan will help you reach your goal, step by step. Think of your plan as a deal you make with yourself.

Make a plan that's realistic. Then you'll feel good about doing the things you've chosen. Read on to see how Pam and Michael made their plans for adding exercise to their daily routines.

What's My Goal for Exercise?

Pam's answer: I want to be more active to keep my blood glucose, blood pressure, and blood fats down.

Michael's answer: I want to be more active so I look and feel better.

☞ What's your answer? _____

_____.

Why Haven't I Exercised Before?

Pam's answer: I didn't exercise before because I thought I was too busy.

Michael's answer: I couldn't play football anymore. I was sad about that and couldn't get started with anything else.

☞ What's your answer? _____

_____.

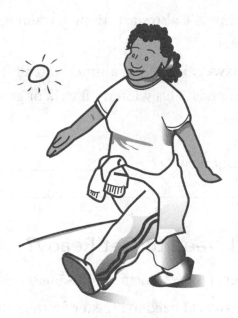

How Can I Work Around This Problem?

Pam's answer: I'll choose activities I can do at home or close to home and that won't take a lot of time.

Michael's answer: I'll talk with my friends about a softball team.

☞ What's your answer? _____

_____.

Here's My Plan: What I'll Do, When, and How Long I'll Do It

Pam's answer: I'll walk 30 minutes three times a week with no more than 2 days between. I'll break this up into two 15-minute sessions or three 10-minute sessions if I'm

short on time. I'll also start strength training at least
1 day a week.

Michael's answer: I'll join a summer softball team and play
with my friends. This winter, I'll walk or go to the gym 3
days a week.

☞ What's your answer? _____
_____.

What Do I Need to Get Ready?

Pam's answer: I need some new walking shoes that fit well.

Michael's answer: I need to register for the softball team.
This winter, I'll need to sign up at the gym.

☞ What's your answer? _____
_____.

What Might Get in the Way of Making This Change?

Pam's answer: The weather might not be good.

Michael's answer: The softball game might be rained out.

☞ What's your answer? _____
_____.

How Can I Get Around the Problem of Making a Change?

Pam's answer: I'll walk inside or do exercises on TV.

Michael's answer: I'll dance with my girlfriend.

☞ What's your answer? _____

_____.

Here's How I'll Reward Myself

Pam's answer: If I meet my goals this week, I'll buy myself a bunch of flowers.

Michael's answer: If I meet my goals this week, I'll go to the movies.

☞ What's your answer? _____

_____.

Go for It!

Now that you have your plan, talk it over with your health care team. Do you need a checkup before getting started?

Remember, motion is the potion! Set your start date!

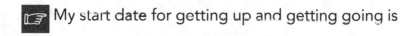 My start date for getting up and getting going is

_____.

—11—

Guidelines for Diabetes Care

Most people with diabetes need to see their health care provider every 3 to 6 months. Before your next diabetes visit, there are things you can do to be sure you're getting up-to-date diabetes care.

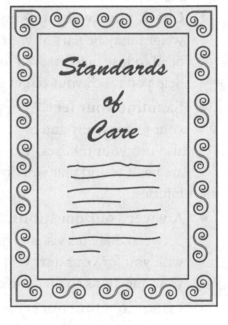

Guidelines from the American Diabetes Association can help people with diabetes live long and healthy lives. Called the **Standards of Care**, these guidelines describe the best diabetes care. Make sure your health care provider uses the Standards of Care to get the most out of your diabetes visits.

At Every Diabetes Visit

If your diabetes health team is following the Standards of Care, at every diabetes visit your team members will:

- **Check your blood pressure.** Your blood pressure numbers tell you the force of blood flow inside your vessels. When your blood pressure is high, your heart has to work harder. If your blood pressure is not on target, work with your diabetes health team. Meal planning, exercise, and medicines can help.

- **Check your weight.** Preventing weight gain or losing weight may be part of your diabetes care plan. If you need to lose weight, even losing 10 to 15 pounds can help you reach your target goals.

- **Examine your feet.** Your care provider will examine your feet visually and by touching them. He or she may also test your reflexes. This exam ensures that your feet are healthy and that you don't have any wounds or injuries.

- **Answer your questions.** When you think of questions between diabetes visits, write them down. Take your list with you for your next visit. Write down the answers to your questions so that you can review them later.

- **Listen to your concerns.** Are you worried about your kidneys or eyes? Talk with your diabetes team about your concerns and worries.

- **Talk to you about ways to quit smoking, if you smoke.** For more on stopping smoking, see page 141 in Chapter 16.

At Least Twice a Year

The Standards of Care suggest that your diabetes care team do this check at least twice a year:

- **Measure your A1C level.** This is the blood glucose check with a memory. Your A1C reflects your average blood glucose over the last 2 or 3 months. It provides the big picture to you and to your diabetes team.

Every Year

The Standards of Care suggest that your diabetes health care team do these checks at least once a year:

- **Check your cholesterol** (koh-LESS-tuh-rol) **and other blood fats.** Your blood cholesterol level may need to be checked more often if you have a problem. See page 167 in Chapter 19 for more on blood fats and cholesterol.
- **Examine your feet.** Take your shoes and socks off when you go into the exam room. Your provider can check for nerve damage or other problems. Your feet may need to be checked more often if you're having foot problems. Learn more about your feet on page 161 in Chapter 19.
- **Check your urine to see if your kidneys are leaking small amounts of protein.** This is called an albumin (alb-YOU-min) test.
- **Check your GFR to see how well your kidneys are filtering wastes from your blood.** GFR stands for glomerular (glow-MAIR-you-lure) filtration rate.

- **Refer you to an eye doctor for an eye exam.** Be sure your eye doctor uses eye drops to dilate your eyes so he or she can see the back of your eye. See page 159 in Chapter 19 for more on eye care.

- **Refer you for diabetes education and nutrition counseling.** You may need a change in your diabetes care plan.

- **Offer you a flu shot.** Every year, ask for a flu shot to keep from getting sick.

- **Offer you a pneumonia vaccine.** You need the pneumonia (NEW-moan-ya) vaccine at least once in your lifetime. If you are 64 years old or older and your shot was more than 5 years ago, get another.

Mama and her health care team work together using the guidelines from the American Diabetes Association. They talk about her A1C results and other lab results. The results help them know how her diabetes care plan is working and about her health.

Things to Do before Each Diabetes Visit

Before each visit with Dr. Wood, Mama does the following things to get the most from her visit:

- **Makes a list of questions.** Dr. Wood and Mama start every visit by going down her list. Questions she sometimes asks are:

- When is my next A1C check?
- Is my A1C target still 6?
- How are my kidneys doing?

- **Makes a list of all of her medicines.** Dr. Wood reviews this list with Mama. To make a list of your medicines, see the My Medicines form on page 195 in Chapter 21, Diabetes Tools.

- **Makes a list of her over-the-counter medicines.** Some over-the-counter medicines can affect your blood pressure and blood glucose. Dr. Wood and Mama review this list, too. The My Medicines form on page 195 also has a section to list your over-the-counter medicines.

- **Takes her blood glucose logbook.** Mama and Dr. Wood look for patterns in her blood glucose to see if her diabetes care plan needs to be changed.

- **Takes paper and pen.** Mama likes to write down what Dr. Wood tells her, so she won't forget.

- **Takes a family member with her.** Mama likes for me or one of her sisters to go with her for her diabetes visit. Mama relies on us for help and support.

- **Learns about new diabetes treatments.** Mama reads the magazine *Diabetes Forecast* each month. She talks to Dr. Wood about new treatments and ways to prevent health problems. Mama feels more in charge of her diabetes care when she's learning new things about diabetes.

Taking Charge of Your Diabetes Visits

You can get the most out of your diabetes visit by being prepared. See the list above of things Mama does for each of her diabetes visits. Also track your targets. Make a copy of the Tracking Your Targets chart at the end of this chapter (pages 93–94) to take with you to your diabetes visits. Work with your health care provider to fill in the blanks and to see if you are meeting your goals.

Or you can call the American Diabetes Association toll-free at 1-800-DIABETES (800-342-2383) and ask for a copy of the Diabetes Outcomes Card, order code 5984-03. It's a wallet-sized card you can use to record your goals and to track your progress. If your diabetes treatment plan isn't working, talk with your provider about changing your plan. Ask your provider whether seeing a diabetes specialist would help.

Tracking Your Targets

The ADA recommends these targets for most people with diabetes. You may have different targets. You can record your targets and results in these spaces.

What to Do	ADA Targets	My Targets	My Results Date	Date	Date
At Every Office Visit					
Review blood glucose numbers					
Before meals	70–130				
2 hours after the start of a meal	Below 180				
Check blood pressure	Below 130/80				
Review meal plan					
Review activity level					
Check weight					
Discuss questions or concerns					
At Least Twice a Year					
A1C	Below 7				

Tracking Your Targets (page 2)

What to Do	ADA Targets	My Targets	My Results Date	Date
At Least Once a Year				
Physical exam				
Cholesterol				
LDL cholesterol	Below 100			
HDL cholesterol (men)	Above 40			
HDL cholesterol (women)	Above 50			
Triglycerides	Below 150			
Kidneys				
Albumin test	Below 30			
GFR	Below 90			
Dilated eye exam				
Flu shot				
Once				
Pneumonia vaccine				

—12—

Diabetes Medicines

People with type 2 diabetes will need changes in their diabetes care plan over time. When you first learned you had type 2 diabetes, you may have changed how much or what you ate. You may have started taking walks to keep your blood glucose in your target range. As time goes on, you may need diabetes pills or insulin or other shots. That doesn't mean your diabetes is getting worse. It just means that your old plan isn't working now. Changing your diabetes treatment plan can help you reach your blood glucose goals.

When Mama and Pam were diagnosed with type 2 diabetes, they were able to keep their blood glucose levels in their target range most of the time without taking diabetes medicines. They lost weight, counted their carbs, walked to be more active, and checked their blood glucose with a meter. They worked hard to keep their blood glucose levels in their target ranges.

When Nathan found out he had diabetes, changing his food and increasing his activity weren't enough to bring his blood glucose down into his target range. He needed to add a diabetes pill to his treatment plan. That did the trick, and Nathan's blood glucose levels were back in his target range.

But as time went by, Nathan noticed that his blood glucose wasn't in his target range as often and that his A1C results were creeping up. Nathan's doctor suggested that Nathan take a second kind of diabetes pill. His current pill works during the night. The new one works after each meal. Taking two pills doesn't mean that Nathan's diabetes is worse. It just means that the pills work even better together than if he were to take only one kind without the other. Together the two pills made Nathan feel better, and his blood glucose and A1C are back on target.

Different diabetes pills work in different ways to keep blood glucose on track. There are many kinds of diabetes pills, and new ones are on the way. Some people with type 2 diabetes take one kind of pill. Others take two kinds of pills or a combination pill because the drugs work better together.

What Kind of Pill Is It?

Diabetes pills work in different ways to keep blood glucose on track. When you get your pills, ask the pharmacist what your pills do and whether they have any side effects or things to look out for. Put a check next to the kinds of pills you take. Then write down the names of your pills, the amount to take, and when to take them.

☐ **Sulfonylureas (SUL-fah-nil-YOO-ree-ahz)**. They help your body make more insulin.

Name:_____

Amount: _____ How often: _____

When to take: _____

☐ **Biguanides (by-GWAN-ides)**. They lower the amount of stored glucose that's released from your liver into your body.

Name:_____

Amount: _____ How often: _____

When to take: _____

☐ **Thiazolidinediones (THY-ah-ZO-lih-deen-DY-owns)**. They lower your body's resistance to insulin. This helps your insulin work even better.

Name:_____

Amount: _____ How often: _____

When to take: _____

☐ **Meglitinides** (meh-GLIT-in-ides). They help your body release a quick burst of insulin when you eat a meal or snack.

Name:_____

Amount: _____ How often: _____

When to take: _____

☐ **Alpha-glucosidase inhibitors** (al-fah gloo-KOHS-ih-dayz in-HIB-it-ers). They slow down the rate at which carbs get into your blood after you eat. If you have hypoglycemia, you must take pure glucose to treat it.

Name:_____

Amount: _____ How often: _____

When to take: _____

☐ **DPP-4 Inhibitors.** They help lower A1C levels without causing low blood glucose.

Name:_____

Amount: _____ How often: _____

When to take: __ _____

☐ **Combination diabetes pills.**

Name:_____

Amount: _____ How often: _____

When to take: _____

☐ **Other pills.**

Name:_____

Amount: _____ How often: _____

When to take: _____

☐ **Other pills.**

Name:_____

Amount: _____ How often: _____

When to take: _____

Don't forget about the My Medicines form on page 195 in Chapter 21, Diabetes Tools. You may prefer to use it rather than filling in your medicines above.

Injectable Diabetes Medicines

There are new diabetes medicines that are used with mealtime insulin to control blood glucose. Talk with your doctor about these new injectable medicines.

Insulin

When Nathan needed surgery on his arm, his diabetes pills weren't keeping his blood glucose in his target range, so he took insulin shots. He needed shots for several weeks afterwards, too. Nathan said, "I was really scared the first time I gave myself a shot. But it wasn't as bad as I thought it would be. At first, I was also worried that once I started taking insulin shots, I'd have to take them forever."

But that's not true. It all depends on what's going on. Sometimes you may need insulin for a short time to keep your blood glucose in your target range.

Nathan used an insulin pen for his insulin shots, but some people use a syringe. An insulin pen has a small needle and a cartridge of insulin that's easier to use.

Some people take both pills and insulin. Robert was having blood glucose readings that were too high in the morning. His team suggested that adding an insulin shot in the evening might help keep his morning blood glucose in his target range. Robert thought it over and decided to try it. He found it was easier to stay in his target range during the day if his blood glucose started out lower in the morning.

Some people with type 2 diabetes need one dose of insulin at their dinner meal or at bedtime, along with diabetes pills. Sometimes diabetes pills stop working, and people with type 2 diabetes start with 2 shots per day of two different types of insulin. Some may go on to 3 or 4 shots of insulin per day.

If you need to add insulin or if you're using insulin now, here are two helpful facts about insulin:

- Insulin can't be taken as a pill. Insulin is a protein and would be digested like other protein foods you eat.
- There are different types of insulin.

Types of Insulin

- **Rapid-acting insulins**, such as lispro (Humalog), aspart (Novolog), and glulisine (Apidra), are the fastest of all insulins. Once you inject rapid-acting insulin, it starts working in about 15 minutes. It works hardest, or peaks, an hour or so after you inject it. It can last 3 to 4 hours. This kind of insulin is designed so you can inject it right before meals. It starts to work about the time you start to eat. By the time your meal is digested and glucose is beginning to move into your blood, rapid-acting insulin is working the hardest at moving the blood glucose into your body cells for energy.
- **Short-acting** or **regular insulin** is also used around mealtime. It takes longer to work than rapid-acting insulin does. You take short-acting insulin about 30 to 45 minutes before you plan to eat. It peaks about 2 to 3

hours later. It can keep working for up to 8 hours. Rapid-acting and short-acting insulin are both "clear" in color.

- **Intermediate-acting insulin**, called NPH, takes longer to work. It provides background insulin but not for meals. It begins to work 2 to 4 hours after you inject it and peaks 6 to 12 hours after being injected. It continues to work for 12 to 18 hours. Intermediate-acting insulin works all day if you take it in the morning. It works all night and with your morning blood glucose levels if you take it in the evening. This type of insulin looks "cloudy" and needs to be mixed before injecting.

- **Long-acting insulins**, such as glargine (sometimes called Lantus) and detemir (sometimes called Levemir), are usually taken in the morning or at bedtime. They start to work about 2 to 4 hours after injection and continue to work for 24 hours with little or no peak. Long-acting insulins can help keep your insulin and blood glucose levels steady throughout the day and night. Long-acting insulins are "clear" in color.

Premixed Insulins

Sometimes insulins work better when different types are combined. Premixed insulins are being used more and more because they are easier to use—you don't have to mix the insulins yourself. If you have poor eyesight or have trouble mixing your insulins, premixed insulin may be helpful. Talk with your health care team if you think a premixed insulin might be right for you.

Insulin Shots

As we saw with Robert, insulin is sometimes needed with type 2 diabetes. Insulin may be taken using a pen, a syringe, or a pump. If your blood glucose levels aren't staying in your target range, talk with your health care team to see if you need to add insulin. Your health care team can help you decide which is best for you.

When you find the right insulin routine, your blood glucose levels will stay in your target range most of the time, and you'll feel better, too.

Selecting an Insulin Pen

Some insulin pens contain a cartridge of insulin that is inserted into the pen. Other insulin pens are prefilled with insulin and discarded after all the insulin has been used. The insulin dose is dialed on the pen, and the insulin is injected through a needle, much like using a syringe. Cartridges and prefilled insulin pens only contain one type of insulin. Two shots will need to be given with two different insulin pens if you are using two types of insulin.

Selecting a Syringe

There are different sizes of syringes. Use the size that is easiest for you to use with your dose of insulin. Also use a syringe big enough that you can read the lettering on the side.

Thin, short needles hurt less. If you're very overweight, a short needle may not work for you. Talk with your diabetes team.

Many people can safely reuse syringes. However, if you are sick or have open wounds on your hands, don't risk reusing a syringe. Keep the needle clean by keeping it capped when not in use. Cleaning the needle with alcohol will remove the coating that helps the needle slide into the skin easily, so don't do that. Keep the needle clean by letting it touch only clean skin or the top of the insulin bottle.

How to Give Yourself an Insulin Shot

If you need to start taking insulin, work with your diabetes health care team to learn how to do it. You'll recall that Nathan started insulin after having surgery. He was really scared the first time he gave himself a shot. But it wasn't as bad as he thought it would be.

Here are the basics for giving an insulin shot. If you have questions, ask your diabetes team for help.

- Decide where to give your insulin shot. You can give your shots pretty much wherever you have enough fat under the skin. The main areas are your stomach, your thighs, and the back of your upper arms. Changing the site where you give your shots is called site rotation. Site rotation prevents a buildup of fat under your skin. Each shot site is about the size of a quarter. You only need to move a finger-width away to give your next shot.

- Most people prefer to give the shots in their stomach. Your stomach is easy to reach. Also, the insulin is absorbed at a steady rate from shot to shot. If you inject in your stomach, don't get too close to your navel, or belly button. The skin around your navel is tougher and makes the insulin action less smooth.

- If you inject in your thigh, use the top and outside area. Stay away from your inner thigh.

- If you inject in your arm, use the outer back area of your upper arm. This is where you have the most fat.

- Some people rotate within only one area, like their stomach. Others give their morning shot in their stomachs and their evening shot in their thigh. Talk with your diabetes team about the best options for you.

● Wash and dry your hands.

● Check the date on the bottle. If it's past that date, don't use it. The insulin is too old.

● Check your insulin before using it.

- Rapid- and long-acting insulins are clear. If that kind of insulin has changed color, is cloudy, or has little bits in it, it is no good. Throw away the bottle.

- Intermediate-acting insulin is cloudy. If you see any large clumps, throw away the bottle.

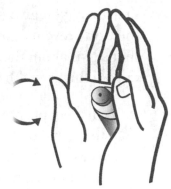

- For those who use intermediate-acting insulin (cloudy): gently roll the insulin bottle in your hands to mix up the insulin. Don't shake the bottle. Shaking can make the insulin clump. Clear insulins don't need to be rolled.

- Work with your diabetes health care team to

  - decide whether to use an insulin pen or a syringe

  - learn how to draw up the right amount and right kinds of insulin in the syringe

  - learn how to dial up the correct amount of insulin if you're using an insulin pen

- When you've got the right amount and right kinds of insulin in an insulin pen or syringe, it's time to give the shot.

- Pinch an inch of skin where you plan to inject the insulin. Pinching an inch makes sure you shoot into fat and not into a muscle. Shooting into a muscle hurts more, and it changes how fast the insulin is used by your body.

- Keep pinching with one hand. With the other hand, hold the syringe like a pencil. Look at the needle to see if it's at the correct angle. The angle depends on how tough your skin is and other factors. Ask your diabetes educator which angle is best for you.

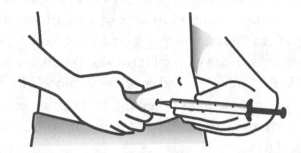

- Gently stick the needle in the skin at the correct angle for you. Press the plunger with your thumb gently and steadily until all the insulin is gone. Check to see if injecting the insulin a little slower or a little faster feels better to you. Then stay with that speed.
- Pull the needle out at the same angle you put it in.
- Press your finger on the shot site for a few seconds to keep the insulin from leaking. If you do have leaking, check your blood glucose more often during the day to be sure it's not too high.
- If you do have leaking often, these tips will help:

    ■ Check the angle of the needle. You may need to straighten the angle a little.

    ■ Push the plunger more slowly when injecting the insulin.

    ■ Count to 10 after pushing in the plunger before removing the needle.

    ■ Check the shot site. If it feels lumpy, choose another site.

If you take insulin and you don't feel well, always check your blood glucose.

- **If your blood glucose is low, first eat something that has about 15 grams of carbohydrate.** Glucose tablets, 1/2 cup of regular (not diet) soft drink or fruit juice, or 1 cup of nonfat (or skim) milk are good choices. Wait 15 minutes, and check your blood glucose again. This is sometimes called the 15-15 rule, see page 73 to learn more about the 15-15 rule. If your blood glucose is still too low, eat another 15 grams of carbohydrate and wait 15 more minutes. Keep following this 15-15 rule until your blood glucose is at least above 70. If it's going to be a few hours before your next meal, have a small snack with carbohydrate. It could be a piece of whole-wheat bread with peanut butter and jelly.

- **Too much insulin.** If you know you took too much insulin, check your blood glucose every 1 to 2 hours and eat extra carbohydrate if your blood glucose is going too low. If you give yourself too much insulin at night, set your alarm clock and check your blood glucose every 1 to 2 hours during the night.

- **If your blood glucose is too high, be more active.** If your blood glucose is often too high, talk with your health care team. Your diabetes plan may need to be updated.

- **Too little insulin.** If you know within an hour that you didn't get all of your insulin dose, give yourself another shot with the rest of the dose. If you don't realize it until later, check your blood glucose level more often during the rest of the day. Watch how many carbs you eat, and be more active.

Taking Care of Insulin

Here are things to do when you're using insulin:

- If you know you're going to use up a whole bottle of insulin within a month, you can keep it at room temperature. It will keep for up to a month if it's not too hot—over 86 degrees.
- If you keep insulin in the refrigerator, warm it up before your shot. Cold insulin can make the shot hurt. Draw up the right amount of insulin into the syringe. Then gently roll the syringe between your hands until it feels warm.
- Don't store insulin in the freezer. Insulin clumps up below 36 degrees and doesn't work.
- Don't store insulin in direct sunlight or in the glove box of your car.

What to Do with Used Syringes

- Be careful when you throw away your used syringes so they won't hurt anyone else. Needles can hurt whoever takes out the trash or picks up the garbage. Check to see if your town and/or state has its own rules for getting rid of used syringes.

Taking Your Medicines

You may take medicines to lower your blood pressure, blood glucose, and blood cholesterol levels. When you're taking lots of medicines, it can be hard to keep track of all of them. Here are some tips that may help you stay healthy:

- Link your pilltaking to something in your day:

  - Always take your medicine after washing your face or brushing your teeth.

  - If you need to take your medicine with food, take it after eating a meal.

  - Use a pill box with sections for each day of the week. The best way yet!

- Ask your diabetes team or pharmacist these questions about your medicines. Write their answers down on a note card or piece of paper, and carry it with you:

  - What are the names of my medicines?
    - Brand name
    - Generic name
  - What's the medicine for?
  - What's the strength of my medicines (such as 25 milligrams)? Milligrams are sometimes written as "mg."
  - How much do I take for one dose?
  - When should I take it?
    - How many times a day?
    - At what times?
    - On an empty stomach?
    - With food?
    - Do I avoid any foods, medicines, or alcohol when I'm taking it?
  - Are there any side effects with this medicine?

- What do I do if I have side effects?
- What if I miss a dose?
- How do I store the medicine?
- How long will the supply last?
- What about refills?

Look at the My Medicines chart on page 195 in Chapter 21, Diabetes Tools. There's also room on the chart for over-the-counter medicines, such as aspirin or cough syrup.

Be sure your health care team is aware of all of the medicines you take. In a paper or plastic bag, bring all your pill bottles, including vitamins and herbal and home remedies, with you when you see your health care team. Or fill in the My Medicines chart in the back of this book and take it with you. Your diabetes team can make sure your medicines all work well together. If you start taking any new pills, they'll check to make sure it's okay to mix them with the pills you're already taking.

—13—

Do You Want to Lose Weight?

Losing weight is one of the best things you can do for your health. Extra weight makes it hard for your insulin to work as well as it could. We all know that losing weight is tough. It takes time and can be a battle. But being overweight is also hard. You may not like the way you look. You may wish you felt better and had more energy. Losing weight can do that for you.

Pam asked how much carbohydrate, protein, and fat would be best to lose weight and keep her blood glucose levels in her target range. Studies have shown that low-fat or low-carb meal plans can help with weight loss. I suggested to Pam that she include foods she loves in her weight loss plan. Pam worked with her dietitian to include foods that tasted good and that kept her blood glucose levels on target. When our meal plan includes the foods we love, we can stick with it.

Losing 10 to 15 pounds can change the way you look and feel. Here are things you can look forward to:

- You'll have more energy.
- Your clothes will fit better.
- Your blood glucose will stay closer to your target range.
- You'll reduce your risk of heart disease and stroke.
- Your blood pressure and blood cholesterol levels will go down.
- You may be able to stop taking diabetes pills or insulin, or you may only need a smaller dose.

Here are some ways you can lose weight and keep it off, even if you've never done it before. Eating regular meals also helps.

Ways to Lose Weight

The bottom line for losing weight is to eat fewer calories than we burn by being more active. We can eat fewer calories by eating less food and less fat.

- **Eat less food.**

  - Try the Rate Your Plate method. See page 14 in Chapter 3 for more information on Rate Your Plate.
  - Eat smaller servings instead of giving up the foods you love.
  - Eat a low-calorie soup or salad before meals. Studies show that people eat fewer calories if they first eat a brothy soup (with lots of liquid and fewer solids) or a large low-calorie salad before their main meal.

- Use a small plate instead of a large dinner plate. This makes it look like we're getting more food. Also, use smaller glasses for drinks.

- Serve smaller portions because we tend to eat everything that we're served. When people are served smaller portions, they eat those portions and feel full.

- Be the last in line at a family gathering. You'll still have food to eat after others have finished eating.

- Eat more slowly, so you're the last one to finish eating. Cut small bites, chew slowly, and chew well. Putting your fork down between bites also helps. Sipping water between bites slows down eating, too.

- Have a fruit or vegetable every time you have a meal or snack. This helps fill you up.

- Go for more salad, vegetables, or fruit if you need a second serving.

- Write down what and how much you eat and drink. Research shows that this is one of the best tools you can use to lose weight. It helps with eating less because you keep track of what you're actually eating. You'll also feel more in control.

- Order the smallest size when eating out.

- Split entrées and desserts with friends and family when eating out. You'll eat less, and you'll save money, too. Or take some home for later or tomorrow's lunch.

- Buy single-serving sizes of snacks, like chips, instead of big bags. You won't be so tempted to eat more than you planned.

- Make your own snack packs by putting pretzels, cookies, nuts, or raisins in a small bag.

- Check serving sizes on food labels. Compare them to the serving sizes you're eating. Often, a can or box has 2 to 4 servings in it, so you could be getting two to four times as many carbs as you think. Review the information on food labeling on page 26.

- Fill up on foods that contain fiber, such as raw or cooked vegetables, fruit, beans, and whole grains. You'll feel full when you finish your meal, and you'll feel full longer.

- Watch out for trigger foods if you're tired, stressed, depressed, or wanting a treat. Trigger foods are foods that trigger you to overeat. Everyone has different trigger foods. It might be salty snacks, white bread, oatmeal, ice cream, or cookies.

☞ Can you think of other ways to eat less food?_____

_____

_____.

☞ Choose one way to eat less food that you think will work for you, and write it here: _____

_____.

If you can eat less food, you'll begin to lose weight, lower your blood glucose, have more energy, and feel good about yourself.

- **Eat less fat.**

  - Fat contains twice as many calories as protein or carbs. Cutting down on fat is a great way to cut down on the calories you eat.

  - Cook lower-fat versions of your favorite recipes.

  - Use fats in small amounts. All fats have lots of calories, even the healthier fats like olive and canola oil, nuts, and seeds.

  - Use nonstick pans and cooking sprays. A quick spray of a nonstick cooking spray in a pan makes it so much easier to use less fat when cooking.

  - Use low-fat versions of foods you like, such as cottage cheese, cream cheese, cheese, salad dressings, mayonnaise, margarine, and sour cream. Full-fat versions of these foods contain more saturated and trans fats, which are not good for your blood vessels and heart.

  - Bake, broil, grill, microwave, or roast meats, chicken, and fish.

  - Eat fried or high-fat foods only once or twice a week.

  - Take the skin off chicken and turkey. Eat breasts and drumsticks more often than wings or thighs.

  - Choose meats that contain the word "loin." They are lower in fat. Tenderloin, sirloin, and loin chops are good choices to save calories and fat. Also, trim any extra fat off meats before cooking.

  - Buy tuna canned in water instead of in oil.

- Try mustard on a sandwich instead of mayonnaise. Or use light mayonnaise.

- Drink nonfat or low-fat milk instead of whole milk. If you're drinking whole milk, take one step and buy 2% milk. In a couple of weeks, take another step and buy 1% milk. Nonfat (or skim) milk is the best choice, but any step you take will save you calories and fat.

- Use 2 egg whites in place of a whole egg in recipes.

☞ Can you think of other ways to eat less fat?_____

_____

_____.

☞ Choose one way to eat less fat that you think will work for you, and write it here: _____

_____.

If you can eat less fat, you'll begin to lose weight, lower your blood glucose, have more energy, and feel better about yourself. You will also have less fat in your blood.

- **Eat regular meals.**

  - Eat some food for breakfast or within a few hours of getting up every day.

  - Eat meals on time. Skipping meals can make you

hungrier and moody and lead to eating more at your next meal. Also, if you take diabetes medicines, skipping meals can cause problems.

- Find the right eating pattern for you. Some people like 3 meals a day. Others like 3 meals and a snack. Some eat 6 small meals a day. Learn what works best for you.

- Plan ahead what you're going to eat. Be sure you have everything on hand that you'll need. Then when you come in late, you'll already know what you're having for dinner. Check out Chapter 4 (page 37) for more on meal planning and shopping.

- Prepare some foods ahead of time. You can cook extra meals on the weekend, first thing in the morning, or the night before. Use a crock pot or a pressure cooker to help you have healthier meals in a short time. And don't forget that freezing meals is another time saver.

- Try to eat about the same time each day. Don't go too long between meals and snacks. This can bring on a binge attack.

- Call a friend, or go for a walk if you're having a craving.

- Check the time, and wait 20 minutes before you eat that trigger food. Many times, you'll be back in control if you hold off for a bit.

☞ My usual meal times are: _____

_____.

☞ My usual snack times are: _____

_____.

☞ Can you think of other ways to eat regular meals?

_____

_____.

☞ Choose one way to try to eat regular meals that you
think will work for you, and write it here: _____

_____.

If you can eat regular meals, you'll begin to lose weight,
lower your blood glucose and blood cholesterol levels, have
more energy, and feel better about yourself.

- **Eat fewer sweets and desserts.**

  - Buy fewer sweets.
  - Buy smaller packages.
  - Share a dessert. Try savoring just three bites of a
    dessert.
  - Drink sugar-free drinks, such as soft drinks and iced
    tea.
  - Use a low-calorie sweetener on your cereal, in your
    coffee, and in cooking, instead of sugar.
  - Buy small juice glasses so you'll drink less juice.
  - Mix juice and seltzer water, and pour over ice for a
    juice cooler. This is a great thirst quencher that cuts
    the calories in half.

- Eat a piece of fruit instead of candy.
- Eat 1 tablespoon of chocolate chips when you need a chocolate fix.
- Try sugar-free or fudge-flavored frozen pops if you think you can eat just one at a time.

☞ Can you think of other ways to eat fewer sweets that will work for you? _____

_____

_____.

☞ Choose one way to eat fewer sweets and desserts that you think will work for you, and write it here:

_____.

If you can eat fewer sweets, you'll begin to lose weight, lower your blood glucose, have more energy, and feel better about yourself.

Nathan lost 10 pounds and has kept it off for 2 years. Nathan said, "Losing weight wasn't the hard part for me. In fact, I've lost the same 10 pounds a dozen times, but every time, I put it all back on plus a few more pounds.

"Even though it was harder for me to lose weight because of my diabetes medicines, I focused on what I could eat. I didn't focus on 'don't eat this' and 'don't eat that.' I still included the foods I love. I just had smaller portions, except for fruits and vegetables. I practiced portion power. I told myself I could have the other half of whatever it was the next day.

"I eat most of the same foods I always did, but I learned to cut back on fat by not frying, using less fat in recipes, and buying low-fat dairy products and salad dressings. I even have low-fat recipes for oven-fried chicken and mashed potatoes made with low-fat buttermilk. I've learned that healthy foods taste good.

"I also use a smaller plate, and my servings look bigger. This really helps with my portion power. I try to drink plenty of water and sugar-free drinks, like iced tea.

"Writing down what I eat and how much I walk every day really helps me stay on track. I reward myself each week by going to a ball game. I have great support from my family, friends, and coworkers.

"I've been able to keep the weight off with a plan and some help. If I can do it, everybody can do it."

Knowing When You're Ready to Lose Weight

When you can put a check next to most of the items below, you're ready to lose weight.

- ☐ I've thought about why I want to lose weight.
- ☐ I think I can do it. I want to do it.
- ☐ I've made a plan for changing the way I eat.
- ☐ I've made a plan for being more active nearly every day.
- ☐ I've thought about how to get around things that have gotten in my way before.
- ☐ I've asked my family, friends, and coworkers for support.
- ☐ I've talked with my health care team about my plan, and I've gotten the help I need from them.

Making Your Plan to Lose Weight

If you're ready to lose weight, these questions will help you make your plan:

☞ Why do I want to lose weight?_____

_____.

☞ What's hard about losing weight for me?_____

_____.

☞ How can I work around these problems? _____

_____.

☞ Who will help me? _____

_____.

☞ What's my plan for losing weight? _____

_____.

☞ What's my first step? _____

_____.

☞ What do I need to get ready? _____

_____.

☞ How will I reward myself? _____

_____.

☞ I'll start my plan on _____ (date).

☞ My weight loss goal is to lose ____ pounds in
1 month. (I suggest to most of the people I work
with to try for 2 to 4 pounds per month.)

☞ My weight loss goal is to lose ____ pounds in
6 months.

☞ My weight loss goal is to lose ____ pounds in 1 year.

How to Track Your Progress

There are many ways to track your success. Choose one or more ways that will be helpful to you.

- Write down what you eat and drink.
- Write down when you eat and drink. If you eat but you're not hungry, write down why you're eating, too.
- Write down the amount of activity you've done. This can be as simple as a hatch mark for 10 minutes of walking. $\cancel{||||}\,|| = 70$ minutes of walking
  Add up the hatch marks at the end of the week to see how you're doing.
- Weigh yourself once a week or once a month. It doesn't matter which one. Keep a log of your weight over time. This will let you see if your plan is working. The best time to check your weight is the first thing in the morning, before you eat or drink anything.
- Use your clothes to measure your success. Can you tighten to the next hole on your belt? Are your jeans fitting better? Can you wear a shirt you haven't worn for awhile?

Don't be tempted by promises of quick weight loss. Watch out for programs that promise you can eat all that you want and still be able to lose weight. Don't be fooled by programs that claim to be easy, quick, or new or that will melt fat away.

Tried and true weight loss methods help you form new habits to lose weight and keep you going until you reach your goal weight. And then those habits will help you keep off the weight that you lost.

—14—

Diabetes and Depression

It's hard to hear that you have type 2 diabetes or prediabetes. It's also hard to live with diabetes on a daily basis. There's never a break from diabetes. There's never a vacation from diabetes. Caring for your diabetes takes time and effort. Sometimes the burden of diabetes can seem like too much to handle. Feeling sad and blue and depressed at times is common for everybody. But if you feel down for 2 weeks or more, talk with your diabetes health care team. You may have depression.

Serious depression is common in people with diabetes. Depression is especially common in women with diabetes. Men get depression, too, but they may be less likely to seek treatment. It isn't clear whether diabetes causes depression or how depression is related to diabetes. It's common for people with prediabetes or diabetes to worry about their health and the effects of diabetes on their lives.

Serious depression is a medical problem, like having high blood pressure or high cholesterol. Depression is not a sign of weakness or failure. This is nothing to feel ashamed about. **The good news is that there are treatments that can help.**

If you have serious depression, it can be hard to get out of bed, do your work, or enjoy anything. You might have trouble being with family and friends or taking care of your diabetes. Counseling or medicine can help you feel better. You'll be able to start enjoying life again. And you'll be able to take care of your diabetes.

Signs of Depression

Watch out for signs that you might need help. Talk with your health care team about help if these things describe you:

- You've been feeling low or depressed for 2 weeks or more.
- You've lost interest in things that used to be fun.
- You've gained or lost a lot of weight.
- You're eating more than usual.
- You're eating less than usual.
- You're unable to sleep.
- You're sleeping too much.
- You're unable to make decisions.
- You're having trouble focusing or thinking things through.
- You feel tired and don't have any energy.

- You're having crying spells or being very emotional.
- You're having trouble making decisions.
- You're thinking about death or suicide.

Signs and symptoms like these are normal after major losses, such as the death of a loved one or a divorce. But people usually start feeling better after a while. People with depression can't trace their symptoms directly to an event. Sometimes it helps to have the support of family and friends. Mama felt sad when she learned she had diabetes. It made her feel down. She didn't like it. Luckily, her family was there to help. She didn't have to go through it alone. Neither do you.

Talk with your friends and family about how you feel and what they can do to help. Maybe you need someone to go with you while you walk. Or maybe you need someone to go with you to your diabetes classes or to your visits with your health care team. But family and friends may not be enough. You may need to talk with members of your health care team, such as the diabetes educator or a counselor.

Living with diabetes isn't easy. While it's normal to be upset sometimes, you don't want these feelings to take over. Here are some tips for coping:

- Write down a list of questions or worries to talk over with your health care team.
- Ask your family and others to support your diabetes care efforts.
- Learn more about diabetes, so you can feel in charge and secure.
- Join a support group.

- Set goals for your diabetes care that you can reach.
- Reach your goals by changing what you do, one step at a time.
- Keep in mind that any steps you take toward your goals will help.
- Talk with a therapist if feelings of depression take over your life.
- Consider volunteering at American Diabetes Association events. You'll get to help other people who have diabetes, and they can help support you!
- Be active. It can help you feel better when you're depressed. Walking, playing with the kids, dancing, or swimming will help lift your spirits.

If you think you are depressed, get help right away. The sooner you get treatment, the sooner you'll feel better.

How Is Depression Treated?

Depression is treated with counseling and medicine, if needed.

Counseling can teach you the skills you need to cope. A mental health counselor can offer a new viewpoint on what's going on in your life.

Medicines for depression help change the way your brain works. Several types are available. Some medicines take several weeks to improve your mood and help you feel back to your normal self.

Your Risk for Depression

Depression can come and go for people with diabetes. Knowing the symptoms and taking action to get help when depression occurs will help you return to feeling like your old self again.

Nathan's Story of Depression

Nathan was really down for a few weeks last spring. Spring is his best time of year, but he wasn't able to enjoy the warm weather or gardening. He couldn't focus on taking care of his diabetes. He felt so down that he didn't bother checking his blood glucose. He didn't care if it was out of his target range.

Nathan ran into a friend who also has diabetes. She said, "Nathan, you don't look so good. Is anything wrong?" Nathan said he was feeling really down. She said, "Nobody likes to talk about feeling down. They worry that people will think they're weak if they admit they're depressed."

Nathan spoke with some of his friends, but it wasn't enough. He talked with his diabetes educator about feeling down and not taking care of his diabetes. Nathan's diabetes educator suggested that he see a therapist.

Over time, talking with the therapist and taking medicine helped Nathan. He told his friends, "Get help if you feel depressed for 2 weeks or more. If you aren't enjoying your hobbies or can't do your work or go to school, get help."

Nathan said, "At first, I thought that feeling down was my fault. But I learned that when you have diabetes, you may have physical changes that can lead to depression. Counseling and medicine helped a lot. I'm glad I got help.

"My depression is gone, and I'm enjoying gardening again. I'm taking care of my diabetes and going to work every day. But I know that because I have diabetes, it may come back. I know what to do if it does. I'll get help a lot sooner."

—15—

Stress and Diabetes

You know that food, exercise, and diabetes medicines all affect your blood glucose levels. But did you know that stress can make your blood glucose level go up?

We feel stressed when problems at home or work put us in a strain. Even happy events, like taking a trip or your son's wedding, can feel stressful. Stress makes it hard to keep your blood glucose on track for two reasons:

- When you're feeling stressed, your body makes hormones that can affect your blood glucose.
- When you're stressed about things in your life, it's hard to take care of your diabetes.

You can't get rid of all the stress in your life, but you can learn to cope with things you can't change.

Mama called me recently saying, "My blood glucose was 275 just 2 hours after my dinner! It's never been that high before. I only had my usual 3 carb choices at dinner tonight.

Do you think my meal plan isn't working anymore?"

We talked about what she had eaten for dinner:

- **1/2 cup black bean and corn salsa**
- **1 corn tortilla**
- Grilled chicken breast
- Tossed salad with light salad dressing
- Iced tea
- **1/2 cup sugar-free pudding**

Indeed, Mama had eaten her 3 carb choices, which are in **bold print** above. I asked her if she felt like she was getting sick with a cold or a sore throat. She said no. Then I asked her if she was worried or stressed about anything.

"Why, yes!" she said. "I was driving today, and a woman in another car started following me and yelling at me. It made me really mad, but it also scared me. It's been on my mind all day. Why would she have done that to me?"

I explained to Mama that her blood glucose might be up because the woman upset her and raised her stress hormones. And those hormones raised her blood glucose. I suggested that Mama check her blood glucose after dinner the next night.

The next night, Mama called and was thrilled. Her blood glucose was back in her target range. Mama said, "I guess my meal plan is still working. My blood glucose was high last night because I was stressed."

When Nathan found out he had diabetes, things were tough. He wanted to make changes to take care of his diabetes.

"There's so much to learn and take care of," Nathan said. "I feel stressed. I don't even want to be with my family or friends anymore."

Nathan talked with his health care team about feeling stressed. He also told them that his blood glucose levels were high and he didn't feel well. He was tired all the time. Nathan wanted to get some ideas about what might help.

Nathan's team suggested he go to a diabetes support group. At his first meeting, Nathan felt out of place. But then someone talked about how hard it was for him when he first got diabetes.

"It helped me a lot to know that he had been stressed, too," Nathan said. "After a couple of meetings, I didn't feel so alone anymore. The people in the group knew what I was going through. I get a lot of help from them. And I've learned that when I help others, it helps me, too."

Are You Stressed Out?

How do **you** feel when you're stressed out? Put a check mark next to the things that are true for you when you're feeling stressed.

- ☐ I get headaches, backaches, or other aches and pains.
- ☐ My muscles get tense.
- ☐ I feel all sweaty.
- ☐ My heart pounds, and I breathe faster.
- ☐ I feel shaky and nervous.
- ☐ I can't sleep.

☐ I feel sad.

☐ I _____.

Feeling shaky or nervous, breathing fast, or having a fast heartbeat can also be caused by low blood glucose.

What do **you** do when you feel stressed?

☐ I eat too much.

☐ I don't feel like eating.

☐ I drink too much alcohol.

☐ I smoke a lot.

☐ I sleep a lot.

☐ I have trouble sleeping.

☐ I have trouble remembering things.

☐ I have a hard time making decisions.

☐ I lose my temper.

☐ I worry about everything.

☐ I don't feel like doing anything.

☐ I pray and meditate.

☐ I get cranky.

☐ I talk to others.

☐ I _____.

Dealing with Stress

- You can't get rid of all the stresses in your life, but you can learn to deal with them. When something goes wrong, don't be hard on yourself. Say to yourself, "I'll do better next time."

- Set goals that you can reach and feel good about.

- Set aside time to relax each day and do something you enjoy. Hobbies, for example, give you time away from daily stresses.

- Exercise is another way to cope with stress, like taking a yoga class or walking around your neighborhood. Try to be active most days of the week.

- Try other new ways to relax. Listening to music, praying, deep breathing, or meditating may help.

- Learning to say no to things you don't need or don't have to do in your life. When we get overwhelmed with too much to do, our stress level goes up every time.

- Some people can relax by taking a bubble bath, lighting a candle and watching it burn, reading, or listening to the rain.

- Talk with family and friends about what you need. They may be able to lighten your stress level.

- Talk with your health care team. They may suggest a support group, counseling, or other services to deal with stress.

—16—

Smoking and Diabetes

You know that having diabetes means you're at risk for certain health problems. But smoking makes your risk even higher for heart disease and eye, kidney, and nerve damage. When you have diabetes and you smoke, it means double trouble. Quitting smoking is one of the hardest things you'll ever do, but you'll be glad you did it. It's truly worth the effort.

Double Trouble

What do diabetes and smoking have in common? They put you at risk for many of the same health problems. Consider the top benefits of giving up smoking:

1. Your blood pressure will go down.
2. You're less likely to have

   - foot problems
   - a stroke

- a heart attack
- nerve problems
- kidney problems

3. Your hair and clothes will smell better.

4. You'll get fewer wrinkles in your face.

5. You'll have healthier gums and teeth.

6. Your loved ones and friends won't be breathing your smoke.

7. You won't have smoker's breath.

8. Your risk for cancer will go down.

9. You'll have more money to spend on other things.

10. If you're a woman, you'll be less likely to have a miscarriage or a stillbirth.

11. If you're a man, you'll be less likely to have **erectile (ee-REK-tyl) dysfunction** (diss-FUHNK-shun), also called **ED** (ee-dee). See page 147 for more about ED.

Have you ever tried to quit smoking? It's hard because smoking is addictive. Your body comes to depend on nicotine. And your mind gets addicted, too. There are lots of hurdles to get over as you try to quit smoking.

Nicotine patches, gum, and new medicines can help. Making a plan can also help.

Are You Ready to Quit Smoking?

Before you quit smoking:

- Think of your reasons to stop, and write them down. Keep your list where you'll see it every day.
- Tell others you'll need their help and understanding.
- Throw away your cigarettes, lighters, and ashtrays.
- Ask a friend or family member to quit smoking with you.
- Join a stop-smoking group.

If you think you're ready to quit, decide how you'll do it:

- Go cold turkey. Quitting all at once works for some people.
- Quit smoking slowly by cutting back over a few weeks.
- Use a nicotine patch or gum.
- Ask your doctor about new medicines for quitting smoking.

Making a Plan

Robert was sick with a cold and sore throat. His smoking made his sore throat and cough worse. He decided he'd had enough. He wanted to try to quit smoking.

His diabetes team helped him make a plan by answering the questions below. Robert's plan worked for him.

Answering these questions will help you make a plan and take the first step toward quitting smoking.

Why Do I Want to Quit Smoking?

Robert's answer: I know smoking means big trouble for people with diabetes.

☞ Your answer: _____

_____.

Why Haven't I Quit Smoking Before?

Robert's answer: Everyone I know smokes.

☞ Your answer: _____

_____.

What Stopped Me from Quitting Smoking Before?

Robert's answer: Smoking helps me handle stress.

☞ Your answer: _____

_____.

I've Tried to Quit Smoking Before. Why Did I Start Smoking Again?

Robert's answer: The addiction was just too strong.

☞ Your answer: _____

_____.

What Can I Do to Keep from Starting Again This Time?

Robert's answer: I'll use a nicotine patch to help with the addiction.

☞ Your answer: _____

_____.

Who Will Help Me?

Robert's answer: I'll join a support group to learn about other ways to handle stress.

☞ Your answer: _____

_____.

What Steps Will I Take to Quit Smoking?

Robert's answer: I'll hang out with people at work who don't smoke.

Your answer: _____
_____.

What Do I Need to Do to Quit Smoking?

Robert's answer: I'll throw away my cigarettes, lighters, and ashtrays. I'll also ask my wife to quit with me. She said she would try to quit, too.

Your answer: _____
_____.

When Will Be the Hardest Times?

Robert's answer: My hardest times will be when I'm stressed or when I'm around people who are smoking.

Your answer: _____
_____.

What Will I Do?

Robert's answer: I'll learn other ways to handle stress in the support group. I'll also tell my friends I'm trying to quit and that I'll need their help.

☞ Your answer: _____

_____.

How Will I Cope with Stress without Smoking?

Robert's answer: I'll take short walks to get rid of my
stress. It works for me.

☞ Your answer: _____

_____.

How Will I Try to Avoid Gaining Weight?

Robert's answer: I've talked with my diabetes health care
team about exercise and meal planning. My wife and I
will take walks after dinner most days of the week. This
will help both of us.

☞ Your answer: _____

_____.

How Will I Set a Date to Quit?

Robert's answer: My wife and I have picked a date,
July 4th, to be free from cigarettes.

☞ Your answer: _____ (date)

How Will I Reward Myself?

Robert's answer: My wife and I will go on a trip. We will be able to afford it. We won't be spending $10 a day on cigarettes anymore!

☞ Your answer: _____

_____.

"In the past," Robert said, "I wasn't ready to quit. This time, I thought about it, made a plan, got help, and set the date. It was hard to do, but I did it. It also helped that my wife quit with me. Having a no-smoking buddy really helps.

"To keep from smoking now," he said, "I've changed some of my routines. Now I take a short walk after lunch instead of smoking. Quitting smoking was one of the hardest things I've ever done, but I'm glad I did it. I'll do whatever it takes to stay away from smoking."

—17—

Sex and Diabetes

Sex is an important part of life and partnerships. But diabetes can affect your sex life. Problems with having sex are not a normal part of getting older and don't happen to all people with diabetes. There is hope. Talk with your health care team about treatments.

For Men Only

Some men with diabetes have **erectile** (ee-REK-tyl) **dysfunction** (diss-FUHNK-shuhn) or **ED** (ee-dee). This used to be called impotence. ED is when a man can no longer have or keep an erection. Over time, blood vessels and nerves in the penis can become damaged. This can lead to ED.

If you have ED, there is hope. There are ways to treat ED that can help. ED is not a normal part of getting older, and it doesn't happen to all men with diabetes. ED can have other causes, such as smoking or prostate or bladder surgery.

It's normal to feel upset if you have ED or some other sexual problem. You may blame yourself or your partner. Some men feel guilty and angry. Others feel like there's no hope. These feelings can make it hard to talk openly with your partner or your doctor. But talking about ED means you're one step closer to getting help.

- There are many ways to treat ED, and more are on the way. If one thing doesn't work, something else might. Talk with your health care provider about your options, such as taking pills to treat ED. If that doesn't work, there are other treatment options.

- Talk with your doctor to see if any medicines you're taking could be causing ED. Some pills for high blood pressure or for depression may cause ED. Pills for stomach ulcers or heartburn also may cause it. There may be other pills you can take. Talk with your doctor before trying any treatment for ED or before stopping any of your medicines.

- Diabetes raises your risk for depression. Depression is a medical problem that's more serious than just feeling a little sad. Depression can lead to ED, and ED can cause men to feel depressed. Talk with your health care team if you feel depressed. Medicines or counseling can help with depression.

If you have ED, it's not the end of your sex life. It can be hard to talk about ED. Even if your doctor doesn't ask about ED, talk about it if you're having problems. Talking about ED is the only way to learn about treatments and get help.

For Women Only

Some women with diabetes have less interest in sex because of depression or frequent yeast infections. High blood glucose levels can make some women feel tired all of the time. Or perhaps intercourse is painful because of vaginal dryness.

If you find you don't enjoy sex anymore, it's normal to feel upset. You may blame yourself or your partner. Some women feel angry or depressed. These feelings can make it hard for you to talk openly with your partner. Don't give up.

Both depression and anxiety can take away your desire for sex. Medicine or counseling can help with both depression and anxiety. If you're feeling depressed or worried for more than 2 weeks, talk with your health care team.

What about hormones? Some women find it hard to keep their blood glucose on track the week before and during their menstrual period. Your blood glucose levels may go up or down because of changes in your hormone levels.

Make a note of the days when you're having your period in your blood glucose logbook. Then look for patterns. Is your blood glucose always high during these days? Talk with your health care team about changing your care plan before, during, or after your period to keep your blood glucose levels on target.

Menopause (MEN-oh-paws), also called the change of life, can affect your blood glucose. As your hormone levels change, you may also have hot flashes or other signs. Talk with your health care team about options. You may need a change in your diabetes plan because changes in hormone levels can affect blood glucose. Also, some women gain weight during menopause. Changing your meal plan or being more active can help keep your weight where you want it.

Here's a list of things you may want to talk about with your health care team. Find a member of your team with whom you feel comfortable. Take a list like this with you to your next diabetes visit:

- Sex is painful for me.
- I don't enjoy sex as much as I did before.
- I'm less interested in sex than before.
- I often have yeast infections.
- I have irregular periods.
- I often feel very sad for more than 2 weeks.
- I often feel very worried.
- I don't feel like I can cope.
- It's hard to stay in my blood glucose target range before or during my period.
- I'm going through the change of life. I would like to know about my options.

Pregnancy and Diabetes

Are you and your partner thinking about having a baby? Diabetes doesn't affect your ability to become a father or a mother. Talk with your health care team if you have questions or concerns.

For women with diabetes who are thinking about becoming pregnant, start working with your health care team well before you get pregnant. Use a safe form of birth control while you're working on your diabetes control. Have your A1C, blood pressure, heart, kidneys, nerves, and eyes checked. See your dietitian to review your meal plan. Talk with your team about how being pregnant will affect your long-term health. If you take diabetes pills, you may need to switch to insulin to protect your baby. You may be referred to a special diabetes and pregnancy team.

You will keep yourself and your baby healthy and safe if you keep your blood glucose in your target range before you get pregnant and until the baby arrives. That will lower your chances of having a premature baby or a baby who's larger than normal. You'll also lower the risk of having a baby with birth defects by keeping your blood glucose close to normal in the first weeks of pregnancy.

If you take medications for your blood pressure, such as ACE inhibitors or angiotensin-receptor blockers (ARBs), or for your cholesterol, such as statins, you may need to stop taking them before you get pregnant. Be sure to discuss the medications you take with your health care provider if you are considering having a baby.

Today, more women with diabetes are able to have healthy babies. With planning and hard work, you can, too.

Birth Control and Diabetes

If you don't want to get pregnant, you'll need to use some kind of birth control. Even if you don't have regular periods, you can still get pregnant. Most birth control methods are safe for women with diabetes. Talk with your health care team about birth control options.

—18—

Alcohol and Diabetes

If you have type 2 diabetes, you may wonder about drinking alcohol. Alcohol can lower or raise your blood glucose. That sounds confusing. The effect of alcohol on blood glucose depends on how much alcohol you drink and if you drink the alcohol with food.

Guidelines for Drinking Alcohol with Type 2 Diabetes

For people with type 2 diabetes, here are some guidelines for drinking alcohol safely:

- Discuss your alcohol-drinking habits with your diabetes health care team.
- Drink alcohol only if your blood glucose levels are in your target range most of the time.

- Limit alcohol to 1 drink or fewer a day if you're a woman. The limit is 2 drinks a day if you're a man. One drink is equal to

  - 12 ounces of beer
  - 5 ounces of wine
  - 1 1/2 ounces of distilled spirits, such as scotch or bourbon.

- Always have a meal or snack that contains carbohydrates when you drink alcohol in order to reduce your risk of low blood glucose, if you take insulin or a diabetes pill that increases your insulin level. Treat alcohol as an addition to your meal or snack. No food needs to be skipped.

- Alcohol makes it harder to know if you have low blood glucose. Drink with a friend or someone who knows you have diabetes and who can treat low blood glucose.

- Alcohol can lower your blood glucose for up to 24 hours after drinking, so be sure to check your blood glucose levels more often when you drink alcohol.

- Mix alcohol with water, club soda, seltzer, or diet drinks. Try a wine spritzer that is made with wine and club soda rather than a sweet wine cooler.

- Stay away from sweet wines, liqueurs, and sweet mixed drinks, such as margaritas. A 1/2 cup or 4 ounces of a margarita mix contains about 2 carbs or 30 grams of carbohydrate.

- Avoid alcohol if you're pregnant or if you've abused alcohol in the past.

- Avoid alcohol if you have other medical problems. Alcohol can make some problems worse.

- Check your medicine bottles to see if the labels say to avoid alcohol.

- Check with your diabetes team if you have questions about drinking alcohol.

Robert's Happy Hour

Robert went out for a beer with his friends after work on a Friday night. There weren't any pretzels on the table like there usually were. They were having a good time and ordered a second round of beers. Tom, one of Robert's friends, noticed that Robert was starting to sweat and seemed confused. Tom said, "Robert, I think your blood glucose is low. Let's all order some sandwiches." After eating the sandwich, Robert felt better.

Robert said, "Thanks, Tom! I needed your help. My blood glucose was low, and I think the beers made it hard for me to know it."

—19—

Long-Term Diabetes Problems

You may be worried about getting long-term diabetes problems, called diabetes complications. Mama was worried about diabetes problems when she found out she had diabetes. She knew all about diabetes problems from her sister, Carla. My patient Michael worried about diabetes problems, too. He knew about the problems his grandparents had from diabetes. Lots of people with diabetes feel this way.

So, what are diabetes problems, and what causes them? Too much glucose in the blood for a long time can cause diabetes problems with your:

- eyes
- feet
- heart and blood vessels
- kidneys
- nervous system
- sex life

- skin
- tooth and gums

See the sections below for more about each kind of problem.

Will you have diabetes problems? You may have one or more diabetes problems or none at all. **The good news is that you can put off or prevent diabetes problems.** The key actions you can take right now to protect yourself from diabetes problems are:

- Keep blood glucose, blood pressure, and blood fats in your target ranges. Studies have shown time and again how important this is.
- Ask your health care team for help with quitting smoking, if you do smoke.
- Stay in contact with your diabetes health care team so that any problems can be found early and treated.

Now let's look at the problems of diabetes one at a time.

Eye Problems

People with diabetes can have eye problems, also called retinopathy (REH-tih-NOP-uh-thee). High blood glucose and high blood pressure can damage your eyes. Carlos is sad about losing his eyesight from type 2 diabetes. Carlos says, "Do what your health care team tells you. I wouldn't be blind if I had taken care of my diabetes. I wish I had a second chance. I'd work with my diabetes team and take care of my diabetes."

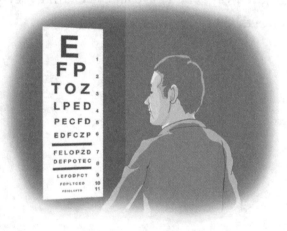

At first, there may not be any warning signs of diabetes eye problems. Later on, there may be changes in your eyesight, such as double vision, floating spots, or flashing lights, or you may have trouble seeing.

But you can delay or prevent eye problems by having an eye exam every year. Have an eye exam more often if you're having eye problems. Be sure your eye doctor uses eye drops to dilate your pupils. By dilating your pupils, the doctor can see the back of your eye and check for problems. This is called a dilated eye exam. Also try to keep your blood glucose and blood pressure in your target ranges to protect your eyes.

If you have an eye problem, your vision might be affected forever if you don't get treated. There are ways to treat diabetic eye problems. Most blindness in people with diabetes can be prevented if it is treated early. Your doctor can use laser therapy to help protect your eyes if you have a problem. A beam of light is aimed through the pupil of your eye to seal weak places in the small blood vessels of your eye.

If you've just been told you have type 2 diabetes, talk to your health care team about referring you to an eye doctor right away. Then have an eye exam every year. Your eyesight is worth it.

Foot Problems

Bill worked in retail and sold shoes. He spent a lot of time on his feet. By the end of the day, his feet would get really tired. Bill said, "Then I got a problem. Even when my feet should have been hurting, I didn't feel a thing. I needed the pain to tell me when I had a problem. But after 20 years with diabetes, my feet didn't feel pain, heat, or cold.

"During a shoe sale at the store, I bought a new pair of shoes and wore them all day. I got a blister but didn't feel it. Before I noticed, the blister had turned into a nasty ulcer.

"One morning after my shower, I saw the ulcer. I went to the doctor right away. I had to go to the hospital for a few days and take antibiotics.

"If I'd let that ulcer go untreated, I might have lost my foot. That's what happened to my Uncle Mike. That's really scary. Now I check my feet every night, no matter what."

After people have had type 2 diabetes over time, they may have less blood flow to their feet and legs. Also, nerve damage from diabetes can lead to loss of feeling in your feet. Minor problems can become big problems and take longer to heal.

Here are some things you can do to protect your feet:

- Keep your blood glucose levels in your target range most of the time. Over time, high blood glucose can damage the blood vessels and the nerves that go to your feet.

- Check your feet
  every day. You
  might want to
  check your feet
  after your bath or
  shower or when
  you're getting
  dressed. Look at
  the tops, bottoms,
  sides, and
  between the toes.
  Use a mirror if
  you can't see the
  bottoms or sides
  of your feet. Or
  ask someone to
  check your feet
  for you. Watch for
  these problems:

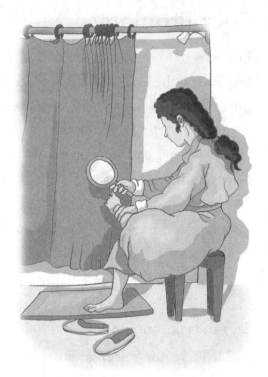

  - Blisters, cuts, redness, swelling, sores, or breaks in
    your skin

  - Corns and calluses. If you have corns or calluses,
    gently use a pumice stone each day. Don't cut corns
    or calluses. This can lead to an infection. Also avoid
    corn removers, but you can use a pad to relieve
    pressure until the corn heals.

  - Ingrown toenails or toenail infections

  - Cold or hot spots, bumps, or dry skin

- Wash your feet with warm water and mild soap. Check
  the water with your wrist first so you won't burn your
  feet.

- Dry your feet well. Be sure to dry between your toes.

- Use lotion if your skin is dry. Don't use lotion between your toes. Infections can grow in dark, moist places.

- Trim or file your nails to match the shape of your toes. Rounded edges help prevent ingrown toenails. If you aren't able to trim your nails, ask someone for help. Your diabetes educator, doctor, or podiatrist (foot doctor) can help with foot care.

- Avoid walking barefoot anywhere, and be careful about wearing sandals.

- Check inside your shoes to be sure there are no objects, like a small stone.

- Protect your feet from hot or cold. Wear shoes at the beach or on hot surfaces. Don't use heating pads or hot water bottles. You can burn your feet without knowing.

Your diabetes health care team can help you prevent foot problems. At every diabetes visit, remind them to look at your feet by taking off your shoes and socks. Ask your provider for a complete foot exam at least once a year and more often if you have a foot problem.

One way to check the feeling in your feet is with a monofilament (mahn-oh-FILL-a-ment). It looks like a piece of nylon fishing line or a bristle in a brush, and it's pressed against the foot to see whether or not you can feel it. Then you and your provider will know if you have numb areas in your feet.

Your provider will look at your skin to check for injuries and may do other checks, such as pulses and reflexes. He'll check for changes in the shape of your foot and look at your toenails.

Most of the time, special shoes and socks aren't needed. If you have nerve damage in your feet, your insurance may pay for special shoes if you need them.

Choose socks without bulky seams at the toes and that aren't too tight at the top.

Bill loves shoes! He sells them, and he likes to wear stylish shoes. He looks for the same things in the shoes he sells as he does in the shoes he buys for himself:

- Style and good fit to prevent blisters or corns. A shoe needs to be long enough and wide enough to allow the toes to wiggle.
- Low-heeled shoes that feel good. High heels put too much stress on your feet.
- Insides that don't have any rough edges that might rub your feet.

Feet keep us moving and enjoying life. Take care of yours every day. You want them to last a lifetime.

Heart and Blood Vessel Problems

People with diabetes are more likely to have heart disease, a heart attack, or a stroke. Their heart attacks can be more serious and can happen early in life to both women and men.

Heart disease happens when blood vessels narrow from a buildup of fat. All blood vessels can be affected. If this happens to the blood vessels to the heart, it can lead to a heart attack. If the vessels to the brain are affected, it can lead to a stroke. If the blood vessels to the legs and feet are affected, it can lead to peripheral (puh-RIF-uh-rul) arterial (ar-TEER-ree-ul) disease or PAD. PAD results in less blood flow to the legs and feet.

The good news is that you can take steps to lower your risk for heart attack, stroke, or PAD. Making wise food choices, being active, and taking medicines, if you need them, can lower your risk and keep your ABCs of diabetes in your target range. So, what are your ABCs of diabetes?

A Is for A1C

You'll recall that the A1C is the blood glucose check with a memory. It tells you your average blood glucose level for the past 2 to 3 months. (See page 61 in Chapter 7 for more on the A1C check.)

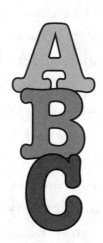

The American Diabetes Association target for A1C is below 7. But your diabetes health care team may set a different target for

A1C		
Diabetes Visit	My Results	My Target
Date:		
Date:		
Date:		
Date:		
Date:		
The American Diabetes Association A1C target is below 7.		

you. Keep track of your A1C results by using the chart above.

Get an A1C check at least twice a year and more often if you aren't in your target range or your diabetes plan changes.

B Is for Blood Pressure

Your blood pressure is always read as two numbers, such as 130/80, and it's spoken as "130 over 80." The first number is the amount of pressure against your blood vessel walls as your heart beats and pushes blood through the blood vessels. The second number is the pressure when your heart rests between beats. High blood pressure raises your risk for heart attack and stroke.

The American Diabetes Association target for blood pressure is below 130 over 80. Your diabetes health care team may set a different blood pressure target for you. Your diabetes team will check your blood pressure at every office visit. You can also check your blood pressure at home or at some grocery stores. Keep track of your blood results by using the chart on the next page.

Blood Pressure		
Diabetes Visit	My Results	My Target
Date:		
Date:		
Date:		
Date:		
Date:		
The American Diabetes Association blood pressure target is below 130 over 80.		

C Is for Cholesterol

Your cholesterol numbers tell you the amount of fats in your blood. There are different kinds of fat in your blood:

- **LDL cholesterol** is sometimes called "bad cholesterol." It can narrow or block blood vessels. Keeping your LDL cholesterol **low** reduces your risk for heart disease.

  The American Diabetes Association target for LDL cholesterol is below 100. Your diabetes health care team may set a different goal for you. Your diabetes team will check your cholesterol level at least once a year and more often if you're having problems. Keep track of your results by using the chart below.

LDL Cholesterol		
Diabetes Visit	My Results	My Target
Date:		
Date:		
Date:		
Date:		
Date:		
The American Diabetes Association LDL cholesterol target is below 100. The target is below 70 if you have cardiovascular disease.		

HDL Cholesterol		
Diabetes Visit	My Results	My Target
Date:		
Date:		
Date:		
Date:		
Date:		

The American Diabetes Association HDL cholesterol target is above 50 for women and above 40 for men.

- **HDL cholesterol** is sometimes called "good cholesterol." It removes fat from your blood and keeps your blood vessels from getting blocked. Keeping HDL cholesterol **high** helps protect you from heart attack or stroke.

  The American Diabetes Association target for HDL cholesterol is different for men and women. The HDL cholesterol target for men is above 40. The HDL cholesterol target for women is above 50. Your diabetes health care team may set a different HDL target for you. Keep track of your results by using the chart above.

- **Triglycerides** are another kind of blood fat that is linked to high blood glucose. High triglycerides raise your risk of a heart attack or stroke. Keeping your triglycerides **low** protects you.

  The American Diabetes Association target for triglycerides is below 150. Your diabetes health care team may set a different triglycerides target for you. Keep track of your results by using the chart on the next page.

Triglycerides		
Diabetes Visit	My Results	My Target
Date:		
Date:		
Date:		
Date:		
Date:		
The American Diabetes Association triglycerides target is below 150.		

Bill's A1C, blood pressure, and cholesterol levels had been running high. He knew he needed to work on taking care of his diabetes ABCs. But it was hard to find time with the crazy hours of his retail job and having time for his family.

He was grilling for a big family party when he had a sharp pain in his chest and felt short of breath. Bill told his wife, Denise, that he didn't feel right. Denise immediately called 911 to get Bill to the emergency room.

Bill said, "They told me it was a heart attack. I'm feeling fine now, and I'm taking the time to take care of my diabetes and my ABCs. I also found out that signs of a heart attack can be different for people with diabetes. Feeling sick to your stomach or short of breath, even without chest pain, is more common during a heart attack in people with diabetes."

Robert woke up feeling very dizzy. He was so dizzy he couldn't get out of bed. He called his son to come over. Robert's son tried to help his dad to the bathroom, but Robert was having trouble walking. Robert's son decided to call 911. He thought his dad might be having a stroke.

What Are the Warning Signs of a Heart Attack?

- Chest pain or discomfort
- Pain or discomfort in your arms, back, jaw, neck, or stomach
- Shortness of breath
- Sweating or light-headedness
- Indigestion or nausea
- Tiredness

If you have warning signs of a heart attack, call 911. Doctors can take steps within an hour of the first warning signs of a heart attack to prevent further damage to your heart.

Tests confirmed that Robert had had a mild stroke. He was treated right away. Now he's back home and doing well.

Both Bill and Robert are working hard to get their ABCs in their target ranges. Check the actions you want to do to take care of your diabetes ABCs:

1. **Change the way you eat by making wise food choices.**
   - ☐ Bake, broil, grill, or roast rather than frying.
   - ☐ Use cooking sprays and nonstick pans.
   - ☐ Choose lean meats and meat substitutes.
   - ☐ Take the skin off poultry.
   - ☐ Buy fat-free or low-fat dairy products, such as nonfat (skim) or 1% milk and low-fat cheeses.

What Are the Warning Signs of a Stroke?

- Weakness or numbness on one side of your body
- Sudden confusion or trouble understanding
- Trouble talking
- Dizziness, loss of balance, or trouble walking
- Trouble seeing out of one or both eyes
- Double vision
- Severe headache

If you have one or more of these warning signs, call 911 right away. Getting treatment within hours can help prevent further damage to your brain.

☐ Eat less fat that raises the risk of heart attack or stroke:

   ○ **Saturated fat** is hard at room temperature. Butter, high-fat dairy products, and fatty meats all contain saturated fat.

   ○ **Trans fat** is found in hydrogenated oils, margarines, and shortening. Trans fats are also found in baked products, such as cookies and crackers. Check the list of ingredients on food labels for hydrogenated fats or partially hydrogenated fats.

☐ Eat fewer high-cholesterol foods, such as egg yolks, organ meats, high-fat meats, and dairy products.

☐ Eat fish that contains fat that protects your heart twice a week. Examples are salmon, sardines, rainbow trout, herring, and mackerel.

☐ Choose good fats, such as canola or olive oil, because they help lower your blood cholesterol level. Nuts, such as almonds and walnuts, also contain good fats.

☐ Work with your dietitian to learn more about choosing heart-healthy foods and the DASH (Dietary Approaches to Stop Hypertension) diet, which may lower your blood pressure.

Put a check mark next to the items above you'd like to try.

2. **Start a new exercise plan**.

☐ Think about an exercise routine you may want to start.

☐ Talk with your health care team about it and what's safe for you.

☐ Make a plan for when and where you'll get your exercise. See Chapter 10 (page 77) for more about making a plan to get up and get going.

Put a check mark next to the items above that will help you start an exercise plan.

3. **Take medicines to lower blood pressure, blood glucose, and blood cholesterol, if you need them.**

• Many medicines can help you reach your ABC targets and lower your risk for a heart attack or stroke.

• Some types of blood pressure and cholesterol medicines can protect your heart. For example, the

American Diabetes Association recommends an ACE inhibitor or an angiotensin-receptor blocker (ARB) to treat high blood pressure in people with diabetes. Talk with your doctor about which of these medicines are best for you. It may take as many as three medicines that work in different ways to reach your blood pressure goals.

- Aspirin may lower your risk of heart disease. Ask your provider if taking aspirin each day is right for you.

People with diabetes are at high risk for a heart attack, stroke, or PAD. Keeping your diabetes ABC numbers close to your targets helps reduce your risk. Talk with your health care team about what you can and will do to protect your heart and reduce your risk.

If you have warning signs of a heart attack or a stroke, call 911. If doctors can see you very soon after the first warning signs, they can prevent further damage.

Review the warning signs on pages 170 and 171 with your family and friends. Tell them about calling 911 to get care right away.

Kidney Problems

Our kidneys filter our blood. They remove things that can harm us and keep things we need. People with diabetes can have kidney problems. This is also called nephropathy (neh-fraw-PUH-thee).

When people have had diabetes for a long time, their kidneys may become damaged. High blood glucose and high blood pressure over time cause damage to the small blood vessels in the kidneys and reduce blood flow.

Early on, there might not be any warning signs of kidney problems. The kidneys work harder to make up for the damage. Later on, the kidneys may become worse. They may not be able to make up for the damage anymore. People may feel very tired or sick to their stomach. Their feet and hands may swell. Their skin may feel itchy.

At Mama's last diabetes visit, her doctor checked her kidneys with these two tests:

- A blood test to measure her GFR. This stands for glomerular (glow-MAIR-you-lure) filtration rate.
- A urine test to measure the amount of protein in her urine. This may be called a urine albumin (alb-YOU-min) check. Protein is not normally found in the urine.

The results of these tests tell you how well your kidneys are working.

Mama's GFR and albumin levels were slightly elevated. Her doctor changed Mama's blood pressure medicine to an

ACE inhibitor. Blood pressure medicines such as ACE inhibitors or ARBs protect your kidneys.

Mama also decided to work harder on lowering her blood glucose to get her A1C to her target. Any lowering of the A1C reduces the risk of diabetes problems, including kidney disease.

If kidney disease isn't found and treated, the kidneys will not be able to clean your blood. This is called "kidney failure." When kidneys fail, the only options are dialysis or a kidney transplant.

The good news is that you can take steps to lower your risk for kidney problems.

- Have a blood test to measure your GFR. The GFR shows how well your kidneys are working.
- Have an albumin test every year to check for small amounts of protein in your urine to see how well your kidneys are working.
- Keep your blood glucose and A1C in your target range.
- Keep your blood pressure on target.
- Talk with your doctor about taking an ACE inhibitor or ARB. These medicines may prevent or delay kidney damage or stop further kidney disease.

Nerve Problems

Diabetes can sometimes cause nerve damage. This is also called neuropathy (new-raw-PUH-thee). The nerves in the feet and legs are the ones most often damaged. Sometimes the nerves in the hands and arms can also be affected.

Nerves that control the stomach, bladder, and digestion can sometimes be damaged. Also, nerve damage causes some people to have problems with sex. For more on sex and diabetes, see Chapter 17 (page 147).

When nerves become damaged by diabetes, some people **feel less** than before. Damaged nerves may not feel pain, heat, or cold.

Robert had lost feeling in his feet. He was out hiking with his buddies. He didn't notice the small stone that had gotten into his shoe. When he got home, he had a bad sore from that little stone he had walked on all day.

If the nerves in your feet are damaged like Robert's, you can't feel pain or an injury. Then a small injury can get worse and become a big problem.

When nerves become damaged by diabetes, some people **feel more** than before. If you feel less or if you feel more depends on what nerves are affected and how they are affected. You may feel burning or tingling. Aunt Carla complained about the weight of the sheets on her feet at night. She also had shooting pain in her legs and feet. These feelings made it hard for her to sleep.

Denise was having low blood glucose a lot, even after eating all of her carbs at lunch or dinner. We checked her food records and logbook and looked for patterns. Her doctor did some tests and found that Denise had nerve damage that was affecting her stomach. She had gastroparesis (gas-TRO-puh-ree-sis). Gastroparesis happens when the nerves to the stomach are damaged or stop working. Food may move too slowly or too quickly through your digestive tract. That's why Denise was having low blood glucose, even after eating her meals. Denise's doctor started her on medicine that helped. We also made changes in her meal plan.

The good news is that there are things you can do to protect yourself from nerve problems.

- Ask your health care provider to check your feet at least once a year to be sure your nerves are still sensitive.
- Check your feet every day for injuries, blisters, redness, or sores.
- Keep your blood glucose and A1C numbers in your target ranges.
- Talk with your health care team if you have any signs of nerve problems. There may be medicines or treatments that can help.

Skin Problems

People with diabetes are more likely to have skin problems. Warning signs of skin problems include:

- athlete's foot
- bleeding
- blisters
- dryness
- infections
- itching

Another skin problem is **acanthosis nigricans** (ak-an-THOH-siss NIG-rih-kans). The skin around the neck or in the armpits appears dark and thick and feels velvety. It can also appear on the hands, elbows, and knees. There is no specific treatment, but caring for your diabetes may cause the changes in your skin to fade.

If you give yourself insulin shots, you can develop rashes, bumpy skin, or pitted skin at injection sites. Some skin problems at injection sites can make it harder for your body to absorb insulin.

The good news is that you can take steps to lower your risk for skin problems.

- ☐ Keep your skin clean.
- ☐ Check your skin every day for dryness and infections.
- ☐ Watch for problems on your feet, under skin folds, and at insulin injection sites.

☐ Keep your A1C in your target range.

☐ Use a mild soap if your skin is itchy.

☐ Use a lotion for dry skin but not between your toes. Infections can grow in dark, moist places.

Tooth and Gum Problems

People with diabetes are more likely to have tooth and gum problems. When you have gum problems, germs work to destroy your gums and the bone around your teeth. Diabetes may weaken your mouth's germ-fighting power. High blood glucose levels can help the germs grow and make the gum disease get worse.

Watch for these warning signs:

- [ ] Bleeding gums when you brush or floss
- [ ] Bad breath
- [ ] Red, swollen, or tender gums
- [ ] Gums that have pulled away from teeth
- [ ] Part of a tooth's root is visible
- [ ] Teeth may look longer
- [ ] Pus between your teeth and gums when you press on your gums
- [ ] Permanent teeth that are loose or moving away from each other
- [ ] Changes in the way your teeth fit when you bite
- [ ] Changes in the fit of partial dentures or bridges

The three main ways to fight gum disease are brushing, flossing, and seeing your dentist regularly. Ask your dentist or hygienist to show you the correct way to brush and floss.

Flossing your teeth cleans away plaque and bits of food from between your teeth and below the gum line. Here are some tips on how to floss:

- ☐ Break off 18 inches of floss, and wind most of it around one of your middle fingers. Wind the rest around the same finger of your other hand.
- ☐ Hold the floss tightly between your thumbs and index fingers. Leave about 1 inch between them.
- ☐ Use a gentle sawing motion to get the floss between your teeth. Never snap the floss into the gums.
- ☐ Curve the floss into a C-shape against one tooth at the gum line. Scrape up and down on the sides of each tooth to remove plaque.
- ☐ Move to a clean section of the floss and continue flossing as it gets worn and dirty. Don't forget the backsides of your rear teeth.

Brushing your teeth cleans the surfaces of your teeth. Here are tips on how to brush:

- ☐ Use a toothbrush with soft bristles and rounded ends. Soft bristles are less likely to hurt your gums.
- ☐ Angle your toothbrush back and forth with short strokes. Use a gentle, scrubbing motion. A toothbrush can only clean one or two teeth at a time.
- ☐ Allow about 3 minutes of brushing to clean all of your teeth well.

☐ Brush the rough surfaces of your tongue to remove germs and freshen your breath.

☐ Get a new toothbrush when the bristles are worn or bent, about every 3 to 4 months.

The good news is that you can lower your risk for tooth and gum problems. You can:

☐ Floss your teeth at least once a day.

☐ Brush your teeth after each meal and snack.

☐ Try to keep your A1C in your target range.

☐ Get your teeth and gums checked and cleaned by your dentist at least twice a year.

☐ Call your doctor if you think you have tooth or gum problems.

Check one or two things in the list above that you want to do to prevent tooth and gum problems.

☞ My start date is _____.

Diabetes Problems: Putting It All Together

You may be worried about getting diabetes problems. As you know from reading this book, lots of people feel this way. **But the good news is that you can delay or prevent diabetes problems.** The key actions you can take right now to protect yourself are:

- ☐ Learn all you can about the early signs of diabetes problems. Getting help right away can keep problems from getting worse.
- ☐ Keep in touch with your diabetes health care team so any problems can be found early and treated.
- ☐ Follow your meal plan that you and your dietitian have worked out. If your meal plan isn't right for you, talk with your dietitian or another member of your diabetes team.
- ☐ Take your medicines as directed.
- ☐ Be active for a total of 30 minutes or more, most days of the week.
- ☐ Don't smoke.
- ☐ Keep your blood glucose, blood pressure, and blood fats in your target ranges.
- ☐ Have a dilated eye exam every year.
- ☐ Check your feet every day for cuts, blisters, sores, swelling, redness, or sore toenails.
- ☐ Take your shoes and socks off to remind your health care team to check your feet.

☐ Have blood and urine tests every year to learn how well your kidneys are working.

☐ Check your skin every day for dryness or infections.

☐ Floss and brush your teeth every day.

What if your doctor says you have a diabetes problem? We all react differently. But here are five steps to help you cope with the problem, make decisions, and get on with your life:

1. **Take the time you need.** In most cases, you will have time to find out your options and decide what is best for you.

2. **Get the support you need.** Look for support from family and friends, people who are going through the same thing you are, and those who have "been there."

3. **Talk with your health care team.** Research shows that talking with your health care team can have positive effects on symptoms and pain. Getting a second opinion may also help you feel more confident about your care.

4. **Seek out information.** When learning about your diabetes problem and its treatment, look for up-to-date information.

5. **Decide on a treatment plan.** Work with your health care team to decide on a treatment plan that best meets your needs.

Research shows that if you are more involved in your health care, you will get better results and be more satisfied.

—20—

What It All Means

Living with diabetes is hard. Learning to live with diabetes takes time and effort. Many of the things we do every single day affect our diabetes and blood glucose levels. The food we eat, how active we are, and how we handle stress all affect our diabetes. The choices you make on a daily basis affect your diabetes and your long-term risk for diabetes problems.

It takes time to take care of your diabetes. Some things may be easier for you, and some things may be harder. For someone else, it may be the other way around.

As you learn more about diabetes and about yourself, you'll learn ways that are easier for you to take care of your diabetes. Make the easier changes first. Take one step at a time.

Learn to lean on your family, friends, and diabetes health care team when you need help and support. Tell them what you need. Is it someone to talk to? Is it someone to walk with? Is it someone to share your problems with? Is it someone to help with shopping? Is it someone to start dinner? Is it someone to cook a healthy meal for you once a week? Is it someone to help with your medicines?

Many of the patients I work with feel guilty a lot. They feel guilty about their diabetes care. They blame themselves when things aren't going right. When their blood glucose levels aren't in their target range, they think it must be their fault. They think they've done something wrong or they haven't done something they should have done. The truth is that sometimes we just don't know why a person's blood glucose is high. Do the best you can each and every day, and let it go.

When you're feeling guilty, think about what could be going on. Are you stressed out? Do you need a change in your diabetes meal plan? Do you need diabetes medicine or a change in your medicine? So many factors affect your diabetes and your diabetes ABCs (A1C, blood pressure, and cholesterol).

Don't feel guilty or blame yourself for being out of your target range. Seek the help and support you need from your diabetes team—your health care team and your family and friends. If you don't think your health care providers are right for you, think about going to other diabetes providers. After all, if you don't like your hairdresser, you go to someone else.

Remember to reward yourself for making changes and making progress. A reward can be as simple as taking the time to do something you enjoy. It can be time to read the newspaper, to watch a movie, to go to the park, to visit a garden, to take a hot bath, or to listen to music. Rewards can also be small purchases. You can buy yourself a flower, a magazine or book, or a CD. A long-term reward could be a weekend trip or a new pair of shoes.

I'll end this book with the way I started it. When it comes to your diabetes care, you are in charge. You choose what and how much to eat. You decide if you'll take your medicines, if you'll check your blood glucose, and if you'll be active. You decide to make and keep your office visits with your health care team.

By taking these actions to care for your diabetes, you'll feel better and have more energy. You can have your share of the good news that long-term diabetes problems can be delayed or even prevented. And taking care of your diabetes can also help to slow or reverse long-term diabetes problems that may have already started.

Take the first step toward your healthier life today!

—21—

Diabetes Tools

This section contains tools that may be helpful to you in taking care of your diabetes:

- A list of carbohydrate foods you can use with carb counting
- A log to keep track of your blood glucose levels
- A chart for listing your medicines
- A calendar for meal planning
- A shopping list
- A list of resources for further learning

Carbohydrate Choices

The number of carb choices that is right for you depends on your weight, your age, and how active you are. Carb choices are also called carb servings. A carb choice is about 15 grams of carbohydrate. Eating 3 or 4 carb choices (45–60 grams of carbohydrate) at each meal and 1 or 2 carb choices (15–30 grams of carbohydrate) for snacks works well for many people. By checking your blood glucose, you'll find out if your meal plan is working for you or if it needs to be tweaked.

You and your dietitian can make a meal plan that fits you. It needs to take into account your likes, dislikes, schedule, and diabetes target goals. Most people need their meal plans reviewed and revised at least once a year. Look on this as your 25,000-mile checkup.

The amount of carbs you eat affects your blood glucose more than anything else you eat, such as protein or fats. The list below shows the size of 1 carb choice.

Carbohydrate Foods List

Starches

Each serving below contains about
15 grams of carbohydrate or 1 carb choice.

1/4	large bagel
1	slice bread
1/2	English muffin, hot dog bun, or hamburger bun
1/2	6-inch pita
3/4	cup ready-to-eat cereal
1/2	cup cooked cereal

1   6-inch tortilla

1   4-inch waffle or pancake

6   crackers

1/3   cup cooked pasta or rice (brown or white)

1/2   cup beans, corn, peas, mashed or boiled potato, or sweet potato

     A handful (about 3/4 ounce) baked chips, pretzels, or low-fat snack crackers

3   cups popcorn

Fruits

Each serving below contains about
15 grams of carbohydrate or 1 carb choice.

1   small fresh fruit (about 4 ounces)

1/2   cup unsweetened canned fruit

2   tablespoons dried apple, cranberries, mixed fruit, or raisins

17   small grapes

1/2   cup fruit juice

1   cup melon

1   cup berries

Milk

Each serving below contains about
15 grams of carbohydrate or 1 carb choice.

1   cup fat-free or 1% milk

6   ounces plain or flavored yogurt (up to 100 calories)

1   cup fat-free or low-fat soy or rice milk

1   cup low-fat buttermilk

Sweets and Desserts

Each serving below contains about
15 grams of carbohydrate or 1 carb choice.

1	2-inch square cake, unfrosted, or small brownie
2	small cookies (2–3 ounces)
1/2	cup light ice cream or frozen yogurt
1	fruit juice bar
1/4	cup sherbet or sorbet

Combo Foods

These foods mix carbohydrates with protein and fats.
They contain different amounts of carbohydrate:

1	cup casserole or chili—2 carb choices and 2 meat servings
1	cup chicken noodle, vegetable, or tomato soup—1 carb choice
1	beef burrito—3 carb choices, 1 meat serving, and 2 fat servings
1/4	of a 10-inch cheese pizza with thin crust—2 carb choices, 2 meat servings, and 2 fat servings
1	medium serving fast-food French fries—4 carb choices and 4 fat servings
1/2	cup coleslaw—1 carb choice and 1 1/2 fat servings
1/3	cup hummus—1 carb choice and 1 meat serving

Free Foods

A free food contains a small amount of carbohydrate and less than
20 calories per serving. You can usually eat as much as you want,
but if a serving size is given, limit the food to three servings per
day to keep your blood glucose in your target range:

1 tablespoon catsup or soy sauce

1 tablespoon fat-free cream cheese, mayonnaise, or
salad dressing

Sugar-free Jell-O

Lemon juice

Mustard

Nonfat cooking spray

1/4 cup salsa

Diet soft drinks

Spices and herbs

Salad greens

1/2 cup cabbage or cucumber

My Blood Glucose Log

Date	Time	Breakfast	Medicine/Comments	Time	Lunch	Medicine/Comments	Time	Dinner	Medicine/Comments	Time	Snack/Other	Medicine/Comments

My Medicines

Medication/Strength	Used for	How Much to Take	When to Take	Notes	Date Started

My Meal Plan
Date:

	Sunday	Monday	Tuesday
Breakfast			
Snack			
Lunch			
Snack			
Dinner			
Snack			
Activity Today			

Wednesday	Thursday	Friday	Saturday

My Shopping List

Vegetables

Canned, Fresh, Frozen

☐ Asparagus
☐ Broccoli
☐ Carrots
☐ Eggplant
☐ Garlic
☐ Greens: collards, turnip
☐ Lettuce
☐ Onions
☐ Peppers: red or green
☐ Potatoes: new or baking
☐ Spinach
☐ Sweet potatoes
☐ Tomatoes

☐ _____
☐ _____

Fruit

Canned, Fresh, Frozen

☐ Apples
☐ Bananas
☐ Blueberries
☐ Cantaloupes
☐ Grapes
☐ Kiwi
☐ Lemons, limes
☐ Oranges
☐ Pears
☐ Raspberries
☐ Strawberries

☐ _____
☐ _____

Whole-Grain Products

☐ Bagels
☐ Bread, whole wheat
☐ Cereals: ready-to-eat or hot
☐ Crackers: low-fat
☐ English muffins
☐ Flour
☐ Pasta
☐ Rice: brown, converted white
☐ Rolls
☐ Thin sandwich rolls and bagels
☐ Tortillas: corn, whole wheat

☐ _____
☐ _____

Meat, Poultry, Fish

Canned, Fresh, Frozen

☐ Beef: loin, round, sirloin
☐ Chicken
☐ Deli meats: turkey, ham
☐ Fish
☐ Pork: chops, loin, tenderloin
☐ Shellfish
☐ Tuna fish: water-packed
☐ Turkey

☐ _____
☐ _____

Dairy Section of Store

- ☐ Butter
- ☐ Cheese: low-fat
- ☐ Cottage cheese: low-fat
- ☐ Eggs or egg substitutes
- ☐ Margarine: low-fat
- ☐ Sour cream: fat-free or low-fat
- ☐ Milk: nonfat (skim), 1%
- ☐ Yogurt: plain, light
- ☐ _____
- ☐ _____

Packaged Foods

- ☐ Beans: canned or dried, black, navy, pinto
- ☐ Frozen dinners: low-fat
- ☐ Pasta sauces
- ☐ Soups
- ☐ Tomato: paste, sauce
- ☐ _____
- ☐ _____

Snacks and Desserts

- ☐ Chips: baked potato, tortilla
- ☐ Cookies: low-fat, wafers, fruit-filled
- ☐ Dried fruit: apples, cranberries, prunes, raisins
- ☐ Jell-O and pudding: sugar-free
- ☐ Ice cream, frozen yogurt: fat-free or low-fat, sugar-free
- ☐ Jam, jelly: sugar-free
- ☐ Nuts
- ☐ Popcorn: low-fat
- ☐ Pretzels

- ☐ Whipped topping: fat-free or low-fat
- ☐ _____
- ☐ _____

Drinks

- ☐ Coffee, tea
- ☐ Drinks, drink mixes: sugar-free
- ☐ Juices: light cranberry, orange, tomato, vegetable
- ☐ _____
- ☐ _____

Condiments

- ☐ Catsup
- ☐ Honey
- ☐ Mayonnaise: low-fat
- ☐ Mustard
- ☐ Olives: green, black
- ☐ Pepper
- ☐ Pickles: low-salt, sugar-free
- ☐ Salad dressing: low-fat
- ☐ Salsa
- ☐ Seeds: sesame, pumpkin, sunflower
- ☐ Salt
- ☐ Spices, herbs
- ☐ Sugar, sugar substitutes
- ☐ Syrup: sugar-free
- ☐ Vinegars: balsamic, cider, red wine, rice wine, white wine
- ☐ _____
- ☐ _____

Other Items

- ☐ Baking powder
- ☐ Baking soda
- ☐ Cooking oils: canola, olive
- ☐ Cooking sprays
- ☐ _____
- ☐ _____

Pharmacy

- ☐ Blood pressure medicines
- ☐ Cholesterol medicines
- ☐ Diabetes medicines
- ☐ Strips for checking blood glucose
- ☐ Other prescription medicines
- ☐ Over-the-counter medicines
- ☐ _____
- ☐ _____

Resources

The **American Diabetes Association** (ADA) is the nation's leading voluntary health organization supporting diabetes research, information and advocacy. Its mission is to prevent and cure diabetes and improve the lives of all people affected by diabetes.

- ✔ ADA local offices are located throughout the nation. To find the ADA office closest to you:

    - Call toll-free 1-888-DIABETES (342-2383).

- ✔ ADA's African-American Initiatives provide programs and outreach efforts in the African-American community. To learn more:

    - Call 1-800-DIABETES (342-2383).
    - Go to www.diabetes.org/in-my-community/ programs/african-american-programs

- ✔ ADA's Education Recognition Program identifies diabetes education programs that meet the National Standards for Diabetes Self-Management Education. To find an ADA Recognized Program in your area:

    - Call 1-800-DIABETES (342-2383).
    - Go to http://professional.diabetes.org/erp_zip_ search.aspx

- ✔ To order ADA books:

    - Call 1-800-232-6733.
    - Go to http://www.shopdiabetes.org

🗸 To find a **Registered Dietitian (RD)** in your area, contact the **American Dietetic Association**.

- Call 1-800-877-1600.
- Go to www.eatright.org/programs/rdfinder

🗸 To find a **Certified Diabetes Educator (CDE)**, contact the **American Association of Diabetes Educators**.

- Call 1-800-338-3633.
- Go to www.diabeteseducator.org/ DiabetesEducation/Find.html

🗸 To get **free information** about diabetes, check out the **National Diabetes Information Clearinghouse** (NDIC), a service of the federal government.

- Call 1-800-860-8747.
- Go to www.diabetes.niddk.nih.gov

🗸 Another great source of **free information** about diabetes is the **National Diabetes Education Program** (NDEP), which is also a service of the federal government.

- Call 1-800-438-5383.
- Go to www.ndep.nih.gov

Index

A

A1C, 58, 61–63, 89, 151, 165–166, 175

acanthosis nigricans, 178

ACE inhibitors, 151, 173, 175

adult-onset diabetes. *See* type 2 diabetes

aerobic exercise, 77

African American, 10

albumin, 89, 174–175

alcohol, 153–155

alpha-glucosidase inhibitor, 74, 98

American Association of Diabetes Educators, 202

American Diabetes Association, 2, 40, 65, 77, 87, 92, 130, 173, 201

American Dietetic Association, 202

angiotensin-receptor blockers, 151, 173, 175

anxiety, 149

armchair exercise, 80

Asian American, 10

aspart, 101

aspirin, 173

B

biguanide, 97

birth control, 152

birth weight, 7

blindness, 159–160

blood fats, 89

blood glucose

  alcohol and, 153

  carbohydrates and, 17–19

  checking your, 57–63

defined, 9–10

exercise and, 78

kidney disease and, 175

logbook, 149, 194

medication, 172

meter, 57–59

pattern, 67

pregnancy and, 151

risk factors, 7

sex and, 149

sick day, 49–50, 52

stress and, 133

target range, 65–75, 158–159, 161

testing. *See* self-monitoring blood glucose

blood pressure, 7, 78, 88, 166–167, 172, 175

blood sugar. *See* blood glucose

blood vessel, 165–173

bronchitis, 54

brushing teeth, 180–182

C

calcium, 27–28

calluses, 162

calories, 27–28, 114

carbohydrate, 16–22, 27–30, 50–52, 81, 154, 189–193. *See also* meal plan; portion power

carbohydrate counting, 16–28, 48

case study

  alcohol, 155

  depression, 132

  exercise, 82–85

  heart attack, 169

  prediabetes, 33–35

  sick day, 54–55

  smoking, 141–146

  stroke, 169

  weight loss, 122

Certified Diabetes Educator (CDE), 2, 202. *See also* health care team

children, 10

cholesterol, 8, 17, 26, 78, 89, 167–173

combination food, 193

combination pills, 99

concerns, 88

condiments, 199

coping tips, 129–130

corns, 162

counseling, 130, 149

D

dairy, 191, 198–199

dental work, 50, 180–182

depression, 127–132, 148–149

desserts, 120–121, 192, 199

detemir, 102

diabetes
    care guidelines, 87–92
    complications, 157–184
    education, 90
    gestational. *See* gestational
        diabetes
    living with, 185–187
    prevalence, 1–2
    prevention, 5–6, 77
    statistics, 4
    tools, 189–193
    treatments, 91
    type 1. *See* type 1 diabetes
    type 2. *See* type 2 diabetes
Diabetes Forecast, 91
Diabetes Outcomes Card, 92
Diabetes Prevention Program, 6
diabetes team. *See* health care
    team; support team
diarrhea, 52
dilated eye exam, 159
dining out, 45–48
doctor visits, 87–92
DPP-4 inhibitors, 98

E

eAG (estimated average
    glucose), 58, 61–63
eating, 13–35, 49–55, 114–121
eating out, 45–48
ED (erectile dysfunction), 140, 147

exercise, 6–7, 71–72, 77–85, 172
eyes, 90, 159–160

F

fast food, 45, 47
fat, 17, 23–24, 26–27, 48, 117–118
fatigue, 149
feeling, 176
feet, 88–89, 161–164
fever, 52
fiber, 28–29, 116
15-15 rule, 73–74, 108
floss, 180–182
flu shot, 69, 90
fluids, 49, 74, 81, 199
food, 13–35
    choices, 28–32, 45–46, 170–172
    combination, 192
    diary, 6–7
    free, 193
    high blood glucose and, 68
    label, 26–28, 116
    liquid, 50–51
    lists, 190–193
    logbook, 115, 125
    packaged, 199
    portions, 14–15, 47
    quick fix, 74
    sick day, 49–55
    soft, 50–51
    trigger, 116, 119

free food, 193
fruits, 29, 191, 198

G

gastroparesis, 177
gestational diabetes, 7
GFR (glomerular filtration
    rate), 89, 174–175
glargine, 102
glucose. *See* blood glucose
glucose gel, 74
glucose tablet, 74
glulisine, 101
glycemic index, 31–32
goals, 82–85
grain products, 198
grocery shopping, 40–43, 198–200
gums, 180–182

H

HDL cholesterol, 8, 168
health care team
    A1C, 58–59
    alcohol, 153–154
    blood glucose levels, 65–66
    care guidelines, 87–92
    complications, eye, 159–160
    complications, preventing, 158
    depression, 128–129
    diabetes, 3–4
    diabetes complications, 183–184
        ED (erectile dysfunction), 148
        exercise, 78, 80–81
        eye complications, 159–160
        foot care, 163–164
        hyperglycemia, 71
        hypoglycemia, 74
        illness, 50, 52–53
        insulin shots, 104–106
        meal planning, 25
        medication, 110–111
        nerve damage, 177
        physical activity, 6
        pregnancy, 151
        sex, 147, 149–150
        stress, 135
heart, 165–173
heart attack, 165, 169–173
heart disease, 165, 173
high blood glucose, 70–72, 108,
    149, 159, 161
high blood pressure, 7, 159
Hispanic American, 10
hormones, 133–134, 149–150
hyperglycemia, 70–72, 108, 149,
    159, 161
hypertension, 7, 159
hypoglycemia, 72–75, 81, 108, 153

I

identification, 81
illness, 49–55, 69

impotence. *See* ED (erectile dysfunction)

ingrown toenails, 162

injectible diabetes medicine, 100

insulin

    about, 100–101

    alcohol and, 153

    care, 109

    defined, 10

    dosage, 108

    pen, 100, 103, 106

    pump, 103

    shots, 103–107

    sick day, 49–50

    syringe, 100, 103–104, 106, 109

    taking care of, 109

    too little, 108

    too much, 108

    types of, 101–102

insulin-dependent diabetes. *See* type 1 diabetes

intermediate-acting insulin, 102, 105–106

iron, 27–28

J

juvenile onset diabetes. *See* type 1 diabetes

K

ketones, 50, 71–72

kidneys, 89, 174–175

L

Latino, 10

LDL cholesterol, 167

lispro, 101

logbook, 60, 91, 149, 194

long-acting insulin, 102, 105

low blood glucose, 72–75, 81, 108, 153

M

maturity-onset diabetes. *See* type 2 diabetes

meal plan

    carbohydrate, 50–51

    complication prevention, 183

    designing a, 25, 190

    eating out, 46

    form, 196–197

    healthy choices, 28–29

    hyperglycemia, 71

    and shopping, 37–43

    weight loss, 113, 119

meal planning tools, 32–35

medical identification, 81

medication
  alcohol and, 153–154
  depression, 130, 149
  diabetes, 95–100
  diabetes care guidelines, 91
  diabetes complications, 172, 183
  ED (erectile dysfunction), 148
  logbook, 195
  nerve damage, 177
  physical activity, 68
  pregnancy, 151
  sick day, 50
  taking your, 109–111
meglitinide, 98
men, 147–148
menopause, 149–150
menstrual period, 149
meter, 57–59
milk, 191
monofilament, 163

N

National Diabetes Education
  Program, 202
National Diabetes Information
  Clearinghouse, 202
Native American, 10
nausea, 51–52
nephropathy, 174
nerve damage, 161, 176–177

neuropathy, 176
NPH insulin, 102
nutrition counseling, 90
Nutrition Facts label, 25–29

O

osteoporosis, 28
over-the-counter medications, 91

P

Pacific Islander, 10
pancreas, 10
pedometer, 7
peripheral arterial disease
  (PAD), 165, 173
pharmacy, 200
physical activity, 6–7, 68, 77–85,
  130
pneumonia vaccine, 90
portion power, 14–24, 47
prediabetes
  case study, 33–35
  defined, 5
  eating and, 13–35
  good news, 2–3
  and insulin, 10
  prevention, 11, 77–78
  risk factors, 7
  statistics, 4
pregnancy, 150–151, 154
premixed insulin, 102

protein, 16–17, 22–23, 198
pump, 103

Q

questions, 88, 90–91
quick-fix food and drink, 74

R

rapid-acting insulin, 101, 105
rate your plate, 14–16, 20, 48,
   114
Registered Dietitian (RD), 202.
   See also health care team
regular insulin, 101–102
resources, 40, 80, 92, 184, 201–202
restaurant food, 45–46
retinopathy, 159
risk factors, 7

S

salad dressing, 47
saturated fat, 17, 26–27, 171
sauces, 47
schedule, 38
self-monitoring blood glucose,
   59–61, 73, 81
serving size, 19–25, 47, 114–116.
   See also portion power
sex, 147–152, 176
shoes, 164
shopping, 40–43, 198–200

short-acting insulin, 101–102
sickness, 49–55, 69
site rotation, 105
skin, 178–179
smoking, 88, 139–146, 158
snacks, 199
socks, 164
sodium, 26–27
sore throat, 51
Standards of Care, 87–89
starches, 190–191
statins, 151
stomach, 176–177
stress, 69, 133–137, 144–145
stretching, 81
stroke, 165, 169–173
sulfonylurea, 97
support team
   alcohol and, 154
   blood glucose testing, 59
   depression, 128–130
   diabetes, 3–4
   diabetes complications, 184
   doctor visits, 91
   eating, 15
   meal planning, 25
   physical activity, 6
   smoking, 145
   stress, 135
sweets, 120–121, 192
syringe, 100, 103–104, 106, 109

T

target blood glucose range,
65–67, 92–94

teeth, 180–182

temperature, 49

thiazolidinedione, 97

tips, 46, 49–50, 129–130

tiredness, 149

tobacco, 88

trans fat, 17, 26–27, 171

treatments, 95–96, 130, 184

triglycerides, 168–169

type 1 diabetes, 9–10

type 2 diabetes
alcohol and, 153–155
eating and, 13–35
good news, 2–3
and insulin, 10
prevention, 7–8, 11, 77
risk factors, 7

U

unsaturated fat, 17

urine, 89, 174

V

vaccine, 90

vaginal dryness, 149

vegetables, 29, 198

vitamins, 27–28

vomiting, 51

W

walking, 6–7

weight gain, 145, 150

weight loss, 6, 78, 88, 113–123

women, 149–150

Y

yeast infection, 149